Self-Seduction

Self-Seduction

Your Ultimate Path to Inner and Outer Beauty

Mikki Taylor

with Photographs by Paul Lange

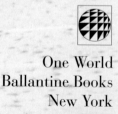

One World
Ballantine Books
New York

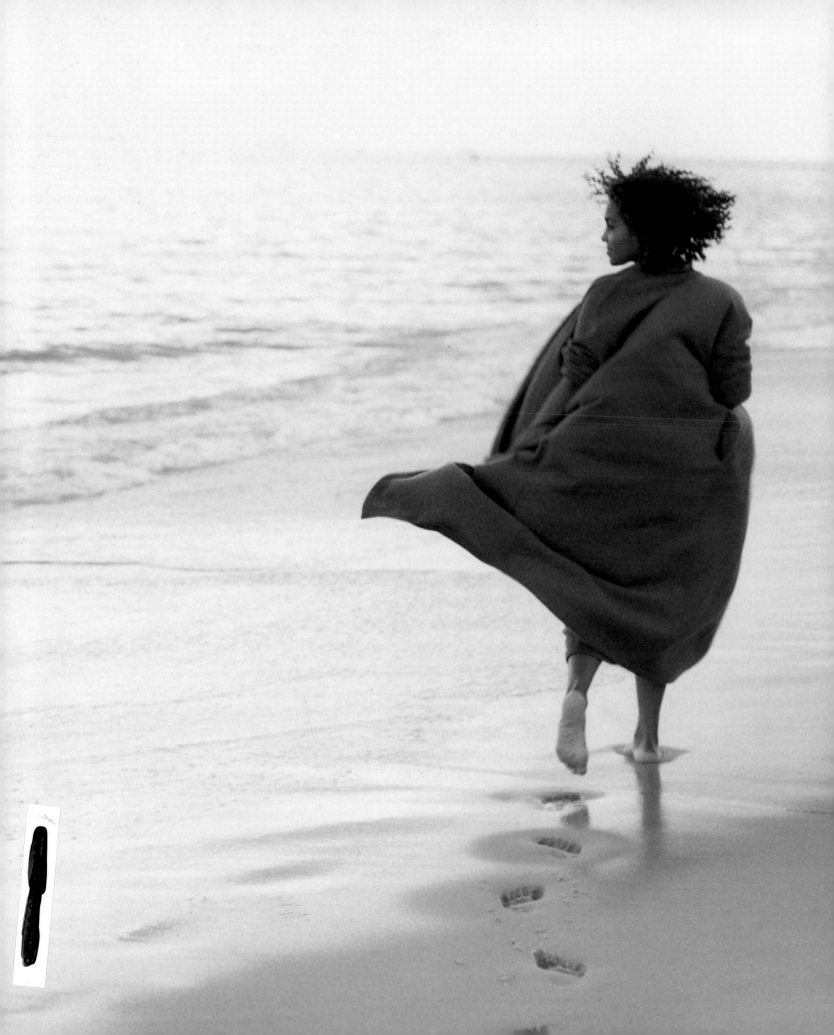

I GIVE THANKS...

To Almighty God, through whom I live, move, and have my very being . . .
my Lord and Savior Jesus Christ for His everlasting love

For my mother, the late Modina Davis Watson, who taught me to fly
and whose wisdom continues to guide me on the journey called life

For Taylor, my darling husband, in whose unconditional love
I am hopelessly lost and forever found

For the jewels in my crown, my beautiful children, Samantha, Philip junior,
and Ms. Ashley, of whom I couldn't be more proud, and my sweetest grandbaby, Modina

For my family, whose love I am more than blessed to have—loving fathers,
Charles and Johnnie, my dear sister, Candace, and my brother, Michael,
and countless aunts, uncles, cousins, nieces, and nephews

And for my brothers and sisters in Christ, friends, and colleagues,
whose encouragement and love I can continually draw on

God is good!

AND PRAISE...

*To my literary agents Michael Broussard and Jan Miller for the kind of belief
and encouragement that turns dreams into reality*

*To photographer Paul Lange, who uniquely captures the soul of a woman
and the depths of an experience, of which I am still in awe*

*To Joel Avirom, Art Director, whose visionary talent brought this journey to life
in ways that take my breath away*

*To S. Raja and the team at Color Edge Labs, for your beautiful work
and generous support of this project*

*To Alkit Pro Camera of New York for your generous contribution and support
of our visualization*

*To Dan Wetuk and Mitchell Broder and the masterful team at Sun Studios, New York City,
for exquisite care and extraordinary support throughout our visual development*

*To Steve Cohen of Space Studio, New York City, for your warmth
and generous help along the way*

*To Timothy White of Whitespace Studio, New York City, for sharing our belief
and supporting our efforts*

To Joe Terrone of EMR Systems Communication for your special efforts and exquisite work

*To Susan L. Taylor, for edifying guidance, encouragement, and wisdom that continues
to push me higher and higher*

To coordinator Sandra "Chief" Martin, for profound support and excellence unequaled

*To style director Pamela R. Macklin, for visionary insight, talent,
and a love that goes the distance*

To Jan de Chabert, for your special encouragement and outstanding contribution

*To Monique A. Greenwood, for such sweet inspiration and the ability to bring out
the best in everyone and everything you touch*

*To Patrik Henry Bass, for your on-point guidance and care—
couldn't have come this far without you, my brother*

To Jay Manuel, for your insights, special support, and unique excellence

*And to the many creative artists who had a "say-so" in capturing the unique beauty
of the women featured herein—you're in a class by yourselves!*

CONTENTS

*I*NTRODUCTION

e are living in an extraordinary age, one when, like no other time before, we are poised to truly pamper and empower ourselves inside and out. Without question, we have the wherewithal to be the women we dream of being and are in hot pursuit of turning our goals into a marvelous reality. In essence, we are here to live out the dream, the future of a sacrificial past handed to us by our elders. And so here, in what has often been labeled "arrival time," one can easily see why our affirmations are centered on "I will" as opposed to "I can" or "I'd like to," because we are more than ready to *own* our lives and celebrate our beauty to the fullest. I can remember a time when my friends and I used to muse about our futures. Why, we'd sit around slapping high fives about what it would be like for each of us when we grew up and established ourselves. Our visions covered the gamut of everything we imagined was involved in the good life, from loving families, to material gains, fab vacations, and a confirmation that we were going to be oh so wonderful to ourselves! Well, little did we know back then that ruling our worlds amid the pressures, unforeseen responsibilities, and seemingly endless to-do lists would all serve to create a pace that would not only throw many of our plans off course but nearly cause us to give up on those confirmations along with it. No one could have told us that even those simple things we were so certain would be a part of having arrived—like time to nurture self beyond those in-and-out visits to get our hair and perhaps our nails done—would continually show up under the category "wishful thinking." And that more often than not the juggling act of trying to succeed at being ourselves, let alone the many extended roles we as women would be called upon to fulfill, would not be so pretty. I certainly know that my vision ended with "and they all lived happily ever after."

Now that I've come of age, I more than know the struggles and the focus required to be all that I can be and not just do all that I can do. I also know that clearly there's a difference, because one leaves me fulfilled and the other leaves me tired and lacking. I know what it's like to want to say "Wait a minute, whose life is this anyway?" when things become overwhelming. But I stopped throwing those pity parties because nobody came!

The dictionary defines *arriving* as "reaching a goal." My girlfriends and I had our visions of what this time would be like, but little did we know that it would require much determination—something God puts in all of us—as well as a strategy to guide and keep it all in place. Nor did we know that reaching such fulfillment would require us to realize what I've come to call *self-seduction*, a sense of loving ourselves in the highest order by committing to what honors us, both within and without—not what moves us to be self-centered, but rather what allows us to become the empowered women we are called to be on all levels. Central to this is the ability to make choices that edify us. When we take charge of our lives and ultimately own our actions, we have truly *arrived*.

These are the outstanding traits that I've observed most about celebrities and women in the know, many of whom are featured in the journey you're about to take. They rule, because this is the wisdom that's at work in their lives; they don't leave anything to chance, but rather take charge with an informed intent and aim for those practices that ensure their beauty—or shall I say their *total well-being*, true beauty in the deeper, substantive sense. From the balance they strive for daily to how they order their spirits and tend their physical and emotional selves, they are owning their lives and celebrating their beauty to the fullest and yet all the while making great strides on the path to self-discovery. I've noticed they also have what I've labeled a *temple management team*—in other words, a coterie of experts that help them keep body, mind, and spirit in a state of fabulosity. Depending on the sister and what season it is in her life, that team can include a variety of experts from, say, a naturopathic doctor, nutritionist, and hairstylist, to a dermatologist, personal trainer, and minister. These women also move through life with a strong support system—a crucial network composed of several sister friends—for they know that when it comes to the subject of their emotional beauty, they have to be careful whom they take their cues from. These and other wise practices help them to live life as totally fulfilled women despite challenge, which is no respecter of persons, titles, or affluence. For sure, they are shaping the lives they desire and the well-being they want to know more of by creating a new script, one day at a time. They more than realize that the key to being their best selves is to tend both their inner and outer beauty, for to have one without the other is to critically sell oneself short. And this, my sisters, is a way of thinking each and every one of us can use. There is no one-plan-fits-all strategy, but rather a call to critical self-examination by looking at where you are and where and how you *want* to be. When 82-year-old body-builder Morjorie Newlin, who's featured in Chapter 5, "Define the Body You Possess," decided to weight-train, she did so because she found out that weight-bearing exercise could offset the effects of osteoporosis and allow her to be strong enough to do the things she desired to do. At 72 she began making this profound investment in her body. Today she competes on an international level, not due to vanity or arrogance or because she has anything to prove to anyone, but because of her determination and passion for owning her life on her own terms. And while she is a size 2, that's totally beside the point, because that's not how she defines her beauty! Rather, Newlin says what's important is that "I'm as independent as I wanted to be and feel really good about myself." For Oscar-winning actress Halle Berry it's essential to have time to meditate—on a daily basis—because after listening to the voices of others all day long, it's important to her to hear her own. To actress Vanessa Williams it means seeing an iridologist, who helps her manage both her inner and outer beauty—in part through juicing and guidance about which foods she should steer clear of, as she knows full well the impact poor eating can have on her overall well-being. For singer Erykah Badu, it means getting what I call that "divine inspired period of healing," otherwise known as sleep, so she can deal; she keeps to the hours of 10:00 P.M. to 6:00 A.M., which allows her some much-needed time for self before waking her young son at 7:00. And then there's the supermodel-turned-cosmetic-entrepreneur Iman, who makes it a point to nurture her physical and emotional beauty by living her life by her priorities, without any guilt. Doing so includes making time for replenishing solitude, whether it's walking to the park for a lovely lunch in the still of the afternoon or spending a half day away from the world at a spa. Ditto for singer Patti LaBelle, who not only directs her life by her own priorities but places a particular emphasis on taking care of herself within so that her outer beauty shines. This she does through prayer, regular colonics, and healing massages. Another sister friend gardens to tend her mind, gain focus, and strengthen her limbs; yet another walks to achieve the same purpose.

In this book you'll find anecdotes, methods, and solution-oriented thinking to help you give new dimension to leading an empowered life. You'll also hear top experts in the fields of health and beauty testify that we can all realize the joys of our desires. One thing's for certain: It all centers on counting ourselves worthy and on knowing, in the words of Dr. JoAnn Magdoff, a psychotherapist in New York City, that it's really a question of allowing yourself to make yourself enough of a priority in your life. I can tell you that managing my life as a wife, busy mother of three, and career woman who's constantly on the road has been a major balancing act. For sure, there were days when I thought there wasn't an extra minute to be had, but I learned to refute that thinking and made it happen by rising early to have that all-important time for self that each of us needs so badly, so I could focus, *style*, and keep on stepping. And when I looked in the mirror one too many times and found that what was on the rise was out of healthy bounds, I decided then and there to stop lamenting my fluctuating weight and stop opening the refrigerator to appease stress. Instead I did the homework, consulted an Ayurvedic expert to understand my makeup and a nutritionist to take the mystery out of healthy eating, and called upon the discipline needed to enable me to have the body I desired. I also made it a point to gain a better perspective on life's challenges by keeping my actions faithful and trusting in my Creator, who the Bible says "neither slumbers nor sleeps." While I couldn't afford a personal trainer, I *was* able to invest in a videotape made by one and was able to use that to reach my goals. Of course, consistently stocking that fridge with the right things and guiding my family on the benefits of this new path didn't hurt either!

You know, it all comes down to "standing in your truth," as Oprah says, and being honest with yourself and becoming more of who *you* are. This is your one and only life, and whatever it is that you want for yourself has to begin with you. And if not now, when? Of all the things I've observed, I've never come across a calendar with an entry for "someday," because it just doesn't show up. So don't even try to reserve a place there—make today *your* day! Begin by doing the inner spiritual work, so key to having and keeping it together, for without this foundation, you'll only be able to deal from a physical perspective in which your sole focus is on how you look. Avoid that trap at all costs. What you want to be is *on purpose*, and let it be known that purpose is what you are about, always! That's when it's for keeps and most meaningful, and that, my sisters, is what you and I can use. When you think about it, what good does a great hairdo, chic makeup, and a closet full of clothes do for you if you're not together on the inside? Absolutely nothing! Keep in mind too this truth, which comes from Proverbs 23:7: "As a man thinketh in his heart, so is he." That's inclusive of us sisters as well. In biblical terms, *heart* actually refers to the mind. So how you see yourself literally defines who you are, for it is the mind that guides our footsteps and propels us into action to develop, enhance, and express our true selves. It is also the place where we behold and judge ourselves. Whatever is revealed in the mind is manifested in the care we give ourselves and ultimately in what we present to the world. Quite simply and amazingly, how you regard yourself inside is another key to true beauty. It is this deeply rooted conviction that allows us to move mind over matter, reach our highest goals, and be the person we all see in our mind's eye. So dare to go there! You know, most stars and sisters who have what I refer to as *celebrité*—that certain something that signals they've got it together long before they utter a word—go to precise lengths to deliver style that is always on point. What I've learned is that it's often based on attitude, one that speaks of a certain confidence and communicates to the world that they know who they are and what's right for them. This kind of confidence doesn't happen by chance; you have to take possession of it deliberately, purposefully. But once you gain it, you get over a whole lot of stuff, for it propels you to live the life *you* want rather than cheating yourself by acting out the one you *think* you should—or, worse yet, just going along with the program.

From there, it's about knowing that the only way for us to step beautifully forward is with a respect for what the ancestors have given us—specifically, those fundamental dos and don'ts for everyday living that affirm our outer beauty stems from within. When I look at the dignity with which first peoples carried themselves, at the loving and devoted time they spent in quiet reflection, and at the rituals of polishing and restoring their temples, I know this is the truth of who we are. It tells me quite frankly that we have an obligation to live our lives to the fullest and in a way that affirms each of us entirely. We can do so by engaging in those rituals that replenish our beauty—from the simplest of acts, such as getting enough sleep and quietude, feeding ourselves only the best foods, and exercising body, mind, and spirit—on a consistent basis.

Thinking back, I can't tell you how grateful I would have been if someone had said to me, "I know the challenges, the desires you want to fulfill, and I'm aware of what a tremendous balancing act it is, but here's how you master it." This, then, my sisters, is the gift I give to you—the path to beauty that leads to being confident, comfortable with yourself, and whole.

—Mikki Taylor

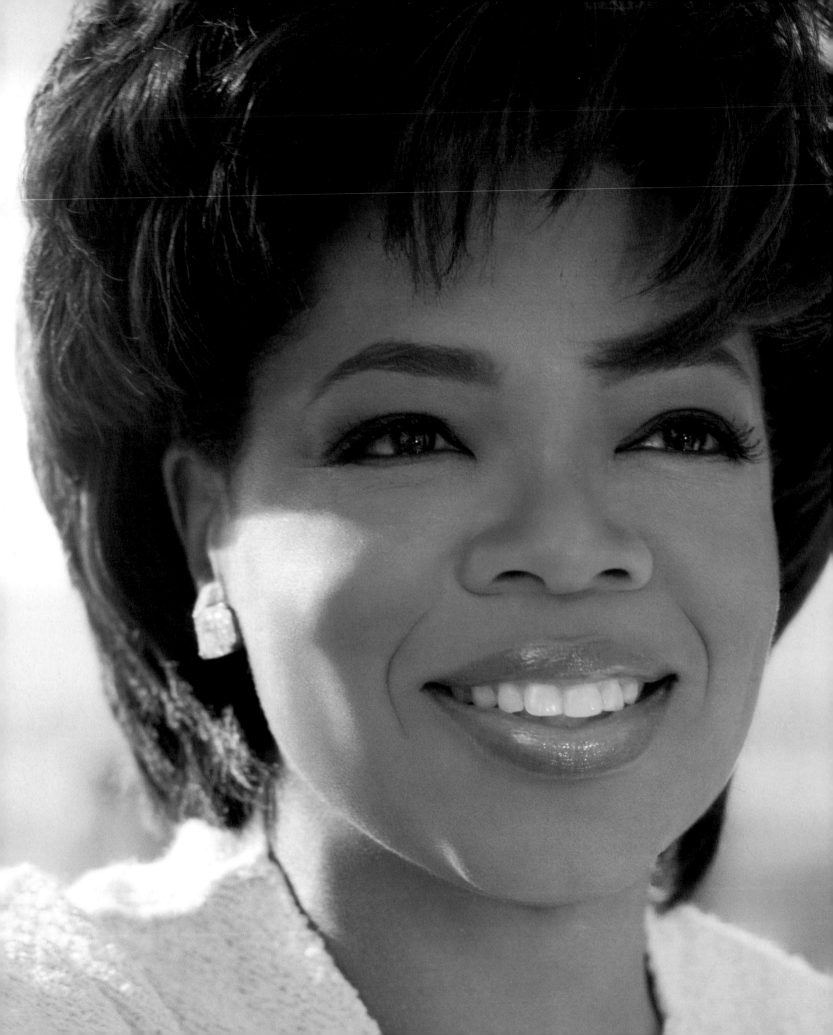

1 ARE YOU LIVING THE LIFE YOU WANT?

"Life is what your Creator gave you for free. Style is what you do with it."

DR. MAE JEMISON,
FIRST AFRICAN-AMERICAN WOMAN IN SPACE

I n my work I've had some grand times and some thrilling experiences. I've dined at the Ritz and pulled my chair up to the table in more celebrity homes than most entertainment reporters combined. Been on the Concorde to Paris and landed in Palm Beach aboard Donald Trump's personal 727. Walked the red carpet at most every glittering award ceremony from New York to L.A., from the Essence Awards to the Oscars. I've worked with the best talent, laid back in all the right spas, gotten cozy at the world's finest hotels, and slipped in and out of more limousines headed to glam-slam occasions in gowns too fabulous to mention. But I didn't touch down on the good life and really start *living* until I got on a rickety old bus with a group of sisters I'll never forget, headed to a retreat for Christian women. Why? I was in search of a necessary truth that eluded me: How does one live the life one really wants, as opposed to living to the life *others* think one should live? I didn't want the snapshot. I wanted the real thing. Don't get me wrong—I absolutely love the work that I do. I'm passionate about beauty and its primary focus, self-discovery, which I think is one of the greatest joys of all. But work is what you *do*, not who you *are*. In fact, it's only one aspect of your life, which, truth be told, is why so many of us crumble when we're forced to walk, because we've allowed it to cross the line from what we do to who we are—but that's another episode. Climbing on that bus, I was clear and ready for the ultimate close-up: I had to get my spiritual house in order, for I believed that was the key that unlocked every other door I desired to open. I'd had more than enough experience going through the motions of life: showing up

PREVIOUS SPREAD:
*Talk show host,
actress, and producer
Oprah Winfrey*

all smiles, talking the talk but not walking the walk, outwardly fabulous but inwardly unraveling. In fact, between the pace I kept, poor eating habits, stress, and an overwhelming to-do list, I was practically writing the script for my own dis-ease. So by the time I took my seat on that bus, I was ready to take the first steps on my path to a new life.

I remember it rained buckets that entire weekend, yet nobody cared about their shoes, their clothes, or their hair but me. It took me almost twenty-four hours to give up, give in, and focus on why I was there. I remember the sisters had a sweet time fellowshipping, a time during which jobs and titles melted away but not their sense of self. What prevailed through the tears of sharing and prayers of petition and praise was an air of gratitude for all they were and all they were going to be in God's perfect will. And more than any state of happiness, which is always dependent upon circumstances, they knew true joy. Their days and their peace were ordered by the Word, so no matter what their personal goals, whether recommitting to the gym or simply vowing to plan for a facial, they were centered and on course. They had purposely stepped away from the busy walk of life to simply nourish their spirits and spend gratifying time in the pleasure of one another's company as well as their own. By day two it became clear to me that for someone who had spent years talking to women about their beauty, I had somehow missed the depth of my own, seeing myself from a mostly superficial perspective as opposed to a richer, spiritual one; not fully taking the time to love myself or to explore the aspect of me that didn't belong to anyone else; never satisfied, wishing I had this or that, equating beauty to a dress size and self-appreciation to how well my body lived up to self-imposed standards. So in the span of three days I got some lessons in living that I will never forget, chief among them a change of heart that caused me to reorder my steps and walk again on higher ground, and to begin to honor my beauty through a deeper sense of appreciation, one that affirms who I am in the eyes of my Creator, who loves me just as I am!

That was my turning point, and since then nothing else has been the same. I stepped out of spiritual poverty and into the rich reality of living the life I desired. My emotional, spiritual, and professional fulfillment became crystal clear to me. In fact, I went on to recognize for the first time that the last of these was really a birthright. You see, I came of age with a respect for beauty and its transforming power that was handed down to me from my mother, the late Modina Davis, who was a wardrobe stylist, hairdresser, and makeup artist to one of the most legendary vocalists of our time, Newark's own Sarah Vaughan. Mother and Sarah had been friends since their school days at Newark's Arts High. In fact, my mother used to do Ada Vaughan's hair (Sarah's mother) during this time, before she eventually went on to do Sass. Their sisterhood was so tight that when Vaughan *arrived*, she purchased the house directly across the street from hers so my mother could be near and took her on the road with her in the 1950s and '60s, traveling the globe for ten years. During this time Mother developed a look for the Divine One (as Sarah was known) that put an image to the voice—from the short and savvy cropped cuts and well-defined makeup to the most gorgeous tulle gowns and flamboyant furs that took your breath away. It was all about perfecting a look that befitted an original icon. And whether Sarah was appearing on Ed Sullivan's show or Jackie Gleason's, wowing the swanky folk at New York's famous Birdland (a hot spot back in the day) or sitting for an album cover or a new set of publicity shots, "Mo," as Mother was known in the industry, had a captivating look for her that would make people sit up and take notice every time. To my mother, presentation was everything. And she gave considerable thought not only to Sarah's image but also to her own. For her, both looking the part and, more deeply, being true to who she was were givens. So she was clear and quite focused when it came to the subjects of beauty and style, and seamless when it came to knowing what worked and what didn't, because for her, these were attributes that stemmed from within.

So it was through my mother's vision that I first learned to dream a world when it came to the subject of style. In fact, to this day I'm so glad that she never made me put my dolls down—I played with them until I was 14—because in reality, I'm still playing with them. Today they're just *living* dolls, and I'm having the thrill of a lifetime helping them discover all the wonderful facets of their beauty. So in truth, I couldn't have done anything else professionally—being a beauty director is as natural to me as the air I breathe. But now I'm ever clearer about the importance of this mission in my journey and the many lives touched through this often life-altering work. And yet, like my mother before me, I have learned to strike a balance and keep my perspective, so that *every* aspect of me is clearly on purpose.

Attending that retreat caused me to finally begin the journey to the woman I desired to be, with some new-life resolutions that would cause me to appreciate my Creator's abundant will for me and to celebrate my beauty to the fullest by living from the inside out, as opposed to the other way around. When you live from the inside out, you are directed from within, your sense of self is on solid ground, and your confidence isn't in the hands of others. When you live from the outside in, you invite chaos and confusion within, you allow yourself to be defined by all the wrong things, and you buy into the untruth that self-esteem is a by-product of achievement. Moreover, you get sucked into folks' opinions of you and other futile stuff that keeps you from appreciating what God has uniquely done in creating you. This is a mind-set that women on higher ground can't use.

This experience also instilled in me the value of spending time with myself to regularly tend my spirit and pamper my *emotional* beauty, something I had largely ignored in favor of the physical. I walked away with tips on how to manage my emotions instead of letting them manage me—in other words, how to check that part of stress that I can control and where to file the rest. This time away also kick-started the process of getting to know myself better, and today I so love the pleasure of my own company! And I've learned to spend it in such solitary ways as gardening, cooking, and working out—why, even the ability to perfectly iron my white linen shirts brings me a distinct joy! I'm also a better wife and lover for it, as well as a pretty cool mom, because I understand more fully the importance of being oneself in life. I'm no longer living outside of my true reality; I know who I am, what I do, and what works for Mikki. I came away altogether motivated to discover my best self, and I've been having the time of my life at it ever since.

People, places, and events are mighty fine, but I've learned that the good life is one that you carve out for yourself, the one you stand firmly in. That in and of itself is the difference between living and existing. Needless to say, I continue to be inspired, and in the process have learned things about myself that make me sit up and take notice. For example, I let stress rule me for years, and it impacted my eating habits as well as altered my body shape and size uncomfortably. No matter what I tried, nothing worked. During that period of dissatisfaction, I started more diets than I care to admit, and the money I spent on unused gym memberships and privileges would have been better off going to charity. It wasn't until I made up my mind that I *wasn't* too busy to do those things that improved the quality of my life as well as my health, like exercise and eat with a well-informed intent, that I lost fifteen pounds for keeps and appreciated it for all the right reasons. I also committed to classes that enhanced my spiritual growth and enabled me to stand firm in life—a difference that I continue to feel and others clearly see.

I don't know where you are in your life, but if you're not living the life you want, then nothing else I'm about to say herein really matters except this: *Living* requires a deeper understanding of who you are and what makes life soar from within. What's found on the journey that is self-seduction are ways to embellish the experience. Many of us are still struggling with this piece, coming close but not fully there yet. Today I continue to honor my resolution to make more self-discoveries, to be more, to live more (not do more), and I want to show you how to have the same appreciation for yourself. What would it take for you to live the life you want? Do you know? If you were told you had a limited amount of time to live, what would you get busy addressing? Is this the point where your inner beauty would become more important than your outer beauty? What is your heart's deepest desire? Only you can answer these questions, but I'll tell you this: Whatever the season of your life, now's the time to respond without hesitation.

For sure, living the life you want is a question of attitude. It's also a question of insight. And I want to push you to dream, to dare to see yourself in the vision, and then don't stop there but get busy making it your reality. This is why the insights of the nation's top experts are present on this journey to guide you. The women found herein, whom I find a continual inspiration, champion this gift from our Creator, otherwise known as life. No matter what life serves them, they've found their joy and aren't about to let it go. They have a clear sense of self and a way of micromanaging their beauty that works, and I want you to know more about their solutions as you define your own. Finally, because I think we all should treat ourselves like celebrities, I'm giving you the all-access pass!

Are You Ready for This?

When we were growing up, my mother continually reminded us that you can't accept anything with closed fists, so I want you to begin this journey by extending your arms and opening your hands, so to speak, in order to fully receive the gifts that are about to come your way. It's time to take stock of what's really important. Let's begin by doing a bit of self-examination about you and how you see yourself as it pertains to your beauty and ultimately how it impacts on living the life you want.

Defining Beauty for Yourself

Just how do you define beauty? Is it centered around the way you wear your hair or makeup? Is it based on your physical characteristics? Perhaps it's more elusive than these qualities; maybe you define beauty as something within. How you characterize it has everything to do with how you see and honor yourself. To me, it's a sense of total well-being, a necessary blend of spiritual and physical health. Moreover, it's about purpose, and we well know that purpose is about more than "How do I look?" Rather, purpose is "What I am about, always!" Contrary to the things we've all been programmed to believe at one time or another, there isn't a standard when it comes to beauty—the very idea of that is an insult to our Creator, who made us all shades, shapes, and sizes—but rather a greater need for self-acceptance. "I define beauty for myself as standing in my own truth and being completely authentic," says talk-show host Oprah Winfrey. Winfrey confesses that she wasn't always so affirmed, however. "I have a picture of myself as a two-year-old next to my bed, and for a long time growing up I used to look at that picture and I wanted it to be different, I wanted a different nose, different lips, I wanted to be somebody else, and now I see that picture and the first thing I say every morning is 'Hi, sweetie.' That is how I think of myself because I have grown into myself. I've grown into my eyes, the fullness of my lips, the broadness of my nose, and I can see my beauty coming on strong." Winfrey says her only regret is that it took her so long to arrive at this station in life. "I'm only sorry that it took me to my forties to get there because I was so consumed until this point with everybody else's idea—none of that exists for me anymore," she adds. This self-empowered sister, who's fully motivated by her own beauty and the joys of living life on her own terms, recalls seeing herself recently on hiatus "buck naked, not a strip of makeup on, hair cornrowed, not a bang, and I just said, 'Hello, sweetie pie!' For me that is growth, what I mean by coming into the fullness of yourself, when you can look into the mirror and what you see just fills you up. I see what God must have seen when He intended this whole thing."

"When you're centered and have it together and love the body that God gave you, you're in harmony, and everything about you radiates that," says Pamela J. Peters, Ph.D., president and founder of the Center for Stress, Pain, and Wellness Management, located in Wilmington, Delaware. This kind of awareness has everything to do with one's state of emotional well-being. "I've been thin and didn't think I was beautiful," says full-figured model Keicia Derry. She's strived to reach the healthy self-image she now possesses by "doing some inner work on self," and fully appreciates her beauty at the size that she is now. Today, beauty for Derry has everything to do with strength and character as well as "being in the light and striving for growth," which she says "just comes with knowing who you are and honoring yourself."

"I believe that getting comfortable in our skin is a decision each sister must consciously make. Like most women of my generation growing up in the 1950s, I wanted to be lighter and have long silky hair," says *ESSENCE* magazine's editorial director Susan L. Taylor. "But what I viewed as beautiful and wanted to look like began to shift the moment I saw the brown and beautiful Dorothy Dandridge on screen in *Carmen Jones*. She looked like many of the women in my family and my Harlem community. She was a goddess!" adds Taylor. What also shaped her thinking was a deeper perspective on Black beauty. "Coming of age in the sixties and learning how all that is African and uniquely beautiful about us was defiled and denied taught me to have reverence for those gifts." This knowledge reached

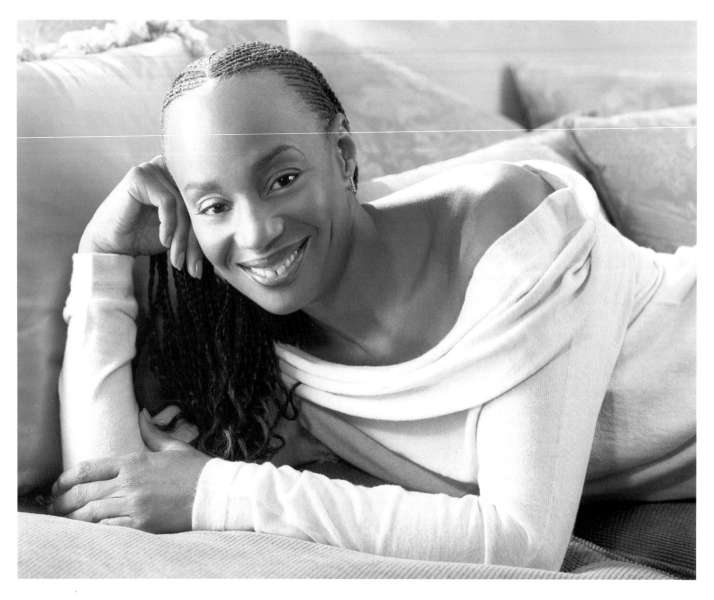

fruition when she began her work at *ESSENCE*. "Joining *ESSENCE* and focusing my efforts and energy each day on putting our beauty on parade made me fall passionately in love with Black womanhood, with our varied looks—our loudness, even—and our power. I just love how we *be* in our many worlds!" says Taylor, whose monthly column, "In the Spirit," teaches sisters how to be their best selves.

Still, in a nation where women of most cultures feel there is a standard of beauty that doesn't include them, celebrating ourselves requires an unwavering awareness. In truth, a poor self-image causes us to act in fear instead of faith. And if we're not careful, we look at what we believe to be wrong with us instead of what is right with God. On the other hand, a positive self-image empowers our actions and motivates us to celebrate all that we are. Says Taylor, "I'm pursuing spiritual perfection. I want to awaken in myself and my sisters fearlessness, compassion, and gratitude for life, for the many gifts God has given us."

ESSENCE editorial director and author Susan L. Taylor

Take a Front-Row Seat in Your Own Life

Is your life full but not fulfilling? Are you good at handling the requests of others but not making any of your own? Do you make time for yourself a priority? Your response to these questions should tell you a lot about where you stand in your own life. Don't feel bad if you answered yes to two or all three of them; just know that a change of heart is in order. As we grow in grace and knowledge, what's important to the journey is for us to begin to count ourselves worthy of being front-row center in our own lives. Do so by taking the time to examine where you are and envision how and where you want to be, and then take this advice from publicist and author of *A Plentiful Harvest: Creating Balance and Harmony Through the Seven Living Virtues*, Terrie Williams, who told me early on, "Make sure you're doing something each week to get there." How many of us have taken the time to examine the deepest desires of our hearts and then really gone about making them happen? Experts say many of us have a list of experiences we want to know but in reality aren't working toward any of them. Far too many of us have put ourselves as well as our desires in the back row, placing everyone and everything ahead of our essential needs. "The most important thing in life is to commit yourself to your own growth and development and to seek your truth, and to finally get a handle on it. If you tend to that, the other things will come to you," says 74-year-old Jacqueline Peters Canon, a holistic counselor and adult-education specialist who lives her life by this belief. Living with this kind of focus isn't easy, but learn to be your own catalyst. Actress LaTanya Richardson Jackson says she came to the conclusion years ago that "you've got to live your life first!" And that requires giving all of yourself a place in your life. The busy, bicoastal, high-profile wife (of actor Samuel L. Jackson) and mother says she's learned to listen to herself and not cover up the way life may be going with "It's okay" (we sisters know we do this so well), but rather to see things for what they are and then act on them, whether it's a question of her body telling her she needs more rest or needing to let some things go.

"We're all longing for the same things: peace, balance, and joy. First we have to train our minds to think differently about ourselves and to want to be gentle, loving, and calm. This is the pathway to living all our dreams. Our challenge is to take the time to envision the life we want to live, to write down our dreams and goals and monitor our time and energy so that they are dedicated to achieving what we desire. Breakthroughs occur when we live with vision and commitment. As Black women, we have learned how to *do*; now we must learn how to *be*," concludes Taylor.

Become Who You Are Meant to Be!

Have you ever made a decision that was out of step with what you wanted in order to please someone else? Ever find yourself at a standstill with your mind focused on your limitations instead of your potential? Have you ever wondered, *What if?* I think there are many women within each of us and that part of the real joy in life lies in discovering as many facets of ourselves as we can. More deeply, the courage to be who you are despite the cost is also so important. Women who possess this quality dress up a world! Once again, it all comes down to "standing in your truth," as Oprah says, and being honest with yourself and becoming more of who *you* are. The more willing you are to embrace the delight, as well as the cost, of being yourself, the more satisfied you'll be. This is your one and only life, and whatever it is that you want to be true of and for you has to begin within.

"You need to be true to who you are and not how somebody else thinks you are," says cosmetic entrepreneur Iman. The modern-day beauty exec, who spends her time discovering the kinds of products that will enhance our beauty, concedes that at 46, she is still "growing up" and finding many revelations about herself as well. "There isn't a day that goes by that you don't learn about yourself. I am better than I was yesterday, but not as good as I'll be tomorrow," she asserts.

A key element of women who have come into the fullness of themselves is an attitude of determination and focus. "I am the author of the only dictionary that defines me," says the outspoken television personality and one of the cohosts of ABC TV's *The View*, Star Jones. For her it's essential to stick to her truth and not conform to that of others, something she sees far too much: "I find that with assimilation we have taken on some of the best and some of the worst." For someone who lives a very public life, Jones also understands how to separate what she does from who she is. "I love playing this over-the-top diva character for people on *The View*, but Star is for the public, Starlet is the private person. In all honesty I can't point to any real failures in my life, and the reason why is because I'm very conscious of who I am."

What also counts is a heady dose of that thing known as perspective. For sisters like Oprah and Susan, that means having their own values and understanding their worth. When you live from this perspective, you always have reason to celebrate, as Oprah points out: "A friend of mine was saying the other day, 'Oh gosh, we're all getting older and there's nothing good about it.' And I said, 'I think it's the greatest!'" Winfrey, who is 49, went on to say, "I'm going to sell the fifties, and I'm going to sell it so that everybody is going to wish they were fifty! It's a time when you know more than you did—you are so centered inside of yourself—you know what you want, you know what you don't want, you know what you will take, you know what you won't take, you are not defined by anyone else's standards!" Says Taylor, "In a world that tells us women that our worth is in looking fine, firm, and forever twenty-two, at fifty-seven, I'm consciously working at loving what I see in the mirror. I'm determined to fall in love with my belly that is less than taut and the sacred space that carried my daughter. I'm working at leaning *toward* the truth, not away from it, and not manipulating it or prettying it up."

As for me, I'm working at keeping the picture fine-tuned. When I became a Christian, as scripture says, old things passed away and I became new. Living this awesome truth causes me to strive to walk in that newness of life that made me whole and in ways that please my Savior. Part of my efforts in this walk of faith includes letting my light shine through good works and a loving spirit, as further emphasis of the truth of who I am in Him day to day. For example, I think of all the gifts the heart has to give, love is chief. Part of my truth is wrapped up in the ability to love others. I really enjoy surprising folks and doing things for them that perhaps they wouldn't do for themselves. These acts of love are essential to satisfying the needs of my heart. Given the life that I live, however, these desires could easily slip through my fingers like reins on a fast-moving chariot, so I have to purposely interject into the plan my need to become more of who I am meant to be spiritually. Now, since I don't believe in wish lists, I keep what I call a "treat list." On that list are goals and things that I'm actively planning for, among them opportunities to do something wonderful for others along my journey. I call it a treat list because the things on this list make my heart jump for joy and move me further along toward the process of succeeding at being myself. I believe God wakes me up every day to do some good. I would hate to have to explain to Him one day that I was too busy.

Becoming who you are meant to be also takes diligence and vision. Long before I ever met Monique Greenwood, author of *Having What Matters: The Black Woman's Guide to Having the Life You Really Want*, I read about her in the *New York Times*. Greenwood was profiled as a serious go-getter, and the article talked about how she'd passed an abandoned house in the Bedford-Stuyvesant section of Brooklyn on her daily cab ride to work and had a vision to turn it into a bed-and-breakfast. Greenwood, who refers to herself as a "bootstrapper," was actually doing more than wishful thinking. She had already begun visiting every bed-and-breakfast she possibly could to learn more about the business, as a dream of hers was to successfully own and operate one in the heart of a renaissance community. The article went on to share her dream come true: the Akwaaba Mansion. Greenwood purchased the majestic eighteen-room mansion and made it happen. When I finally met her, she had come to share her expertise on style and self-empowerment as *ESSENCE* magazine's fashion director. Soon after, she became editor in chief. During her tenure, she pushed women to dream their own dreams and to identify and dispel any illusions that held them back, all the while juggling the sometimes overwhelming demands of being an editor and a business owner, not to mention a mother and wife. Pursuing the woman she was meant to be led to Greenwood relinquishing her role at the magazine to do what she was called to do. She has opened such businesses as the Akwaaba Café, also located in Brooklyn, and another bed-and-breakfast, Akwaaba by the Sea, in Cape May, New Jersey, and is on to fulfilling her desires for more opportunities to host us with the kind of hospitality she delights in. This life change has resulted in more time for self, something this busy sister says she recognizes that she's so "deserving of." For Greenwood, having what matters includes a sense of purpose and a balanced, joyful life, one she has found in responding to the desires of her heart.

The Creator has given each and every one of us gifts that are uniquely ours. Whether we turn them into a thriving business or simply utilize them as a self-fulfilling hobby, we owe it to ourselves to make sure that we get busy doing so and not put this aspect of ourselves on hold. Sometimes we take detours along the way, when headed from where we are to where we need to be. But I can tell you this, detours only prolong the journey to fulfillment. It's better then to step out on faith—albeit one step at a time—toward that which is in your best interest. In the end, you'll always be glad you did.

"So you've got to tell yourself the truth every day, you've got to know when you're pretending, and you've got to stop, because nobody ever reaches what the Creator intended for them to reach as long as they're pretending to be something else. And you've got to get really still, still enough to know the difference between what you want and what everybody else has decided that you want. That's how you find out who you really are, but you've got to get quiet enough to know. And once you've decided and that is coming from the truth of your soul and it's not what anybody else decided that you should be or do, God will rise up to meet you. Everybody told me I wouldn't succeed in Chicago, but I knew that I could tell the truth, I knew that I could be myself. And that's what has helped me the most, to continue to be myself and to search for my authenticity," says Winfrey.

Tend Your Emotional Beauty

Do you take time for self regularly? Do you detox mentally? How often do you reward yourself? Have you fully let go of painful past experiences that may hinder your growth? What do you do to stop the wear and tear on your inner beauty? The answer to questions like these can be tough for we sisters who seldom pull over to the side of the road for a much-needed break. But know that your emotional beauty has a direct impact on your looks as well as your life. And many things affect it, from toxic folks to white sugar! I have well learned the particular perils of the latter, which I am convinced is parallel to a drug. I began to move sugar out of my life about a year ago and have since replaced it with another natural sweetener. To do so, I went on a three-day detox plan, guided by a nutritionist, to help me get over the hump of craving sweet things. By day three I had no desire for any of those goodies that deplete my energy and eventually show up in my attitude with a bit of edge that's not fashionable! I slept better, felt lighter, and was more energized.

I find that taking that necessary time for self impacts my emotional beauty as well. When I don't do so, I'm fidgety, irritable, and oftentimes somewhat resistant to a particular task at hand. I have learned, if nothing else, to hear my own plea for help! This is why I encourage you to give your emotional beauty the attention it deserves. There are a variety of ways to tend it, from taking quiet time to putting back what the world has taken away by giving to others. "Emotionally I know I'm fulfilled when I've given myself unconditionally. My friends nurture me and those I admire, feel the same way about me in return, particularly having known my struggles," says Jennifer Thread McHenry, a fashion buyer and store manager in the Los Angeles area. McHenry, who as a divorced single parent is about the business of grooming her three daughters, ages 7, 9, and 22, to be empowered women, says she's also learned not to be so hard on herself. "It means constantly forgiving myself, because I'm going to make mistakes. And to learn and grow and leave my mind, heart, and soul open in the process," she adds.

In a time where the idea of who's beautiful is constantly changing, letting God assure you of your worth independent of the world's values is also a primer for tending your emotional self. "I wrap myself in a prayer," says Richardson Jackson. The actress says she is so totally *not* what Hollywood is looking for that she's conditioned herself not to get her feelings hurt. "I've also developed a callus from having my parents always telling me that I'm beautiful," she adds. "As we're evolving as a people, it's what you believe in—that's why I never get trapped into feeling I'm not as beautiful as my blond, blue-eyed counterparts," says actress Halle Berry. In fact, when I asked Berry what winning an Oscar meant, she responded, "It said to me that I can do whatever I dare to dream. So that affirmation is the food that inspires me to continue to do more, to be better. What else is there left for me to do? It's inspired me to search that out and not be afraid, because here I accomplished a goal that was just a dream. And it sort of defined that for me, that there is nothing that's unobtainable if you put your heart and soul into it and it becomes a passion in the core and center of your being—that we're powerful people and we can make it happen! I really believe that!"

"I was *colored* and brown-skinned in Mississippi in 1954 and *all* that that means," Winfrey emphatically recounts. "When I left my grandmother to live with my mother, she was rooming with this light-skinned lady named Mrs. Miller, and my mother had already had another child who was also light-skinned, and I, the dark-skinned child, was not allowed in the house. I had to sleep out in the hallway. So when you have that *telling*, nobody has to say 'You ain't the pretty one'—something tells you that you're not. And everything around you says, 'Oh, okay, I got it, it's because I'm the brown-skinned one.' So it has been a long time coming that I can look in the mirror and look at that picture of myself as a little girl and say, 'Hi, sweetie,'" Oprah recalls.

"Throughout my life, emotional pain has compelled me to change my thinking and what I value and give my time and attention to. Today my emotional and physical well-being is paramount to me. Today I *choose* to be loving and kind to myself," confirms Taylor. McHenry concurs and says she makes a point of tending herself at the start of her day through prayer. "I go to the beach and I run about four or five miles and I start off asking God to help me be the best woman I can be: 'Let me be patient, let me be kind, let me be unselfish.' By the end of my run with Him I have settled on different dilemmas, and I leave there strengthened and empowered." Speaking of her emotional beauty, Berry says she's learned a few things: "When it comes down to a spiritual level, when the bottom's pulled out and I find I'm in a valley, I know there's a lesson in this." And so the young actress has learned to take note of experiences that challenge her and to be empowered by them and the knowledge that comes along with them. I've heard the elders talk often about getting those all-important lessons while in the valley, as these are the ones that help you to grow by leaps and bounds. In fact, it is often said that if you miss the lesson, you'll likely find yourself facing the test again!

Tending your emotional beauty requires that you tap into your deepest desires and act on them. If you're a sister who's waiting for that divine-right love to come into your life, show yourself some TLC and use this time to be especially nurturing to yourself. If you're an incurable romantic, let those flowers that you desire show up by your own hand. It tells you that you love yourself enough, that *you* think you're quite special and more than worthy. If you love being stroked, after a steamy bath take body oil and massage yourself. This is the kind of action that feeds your physical as well as your emotional beauty. So don't wait for someone else to find the key to your heart—use it yourself!

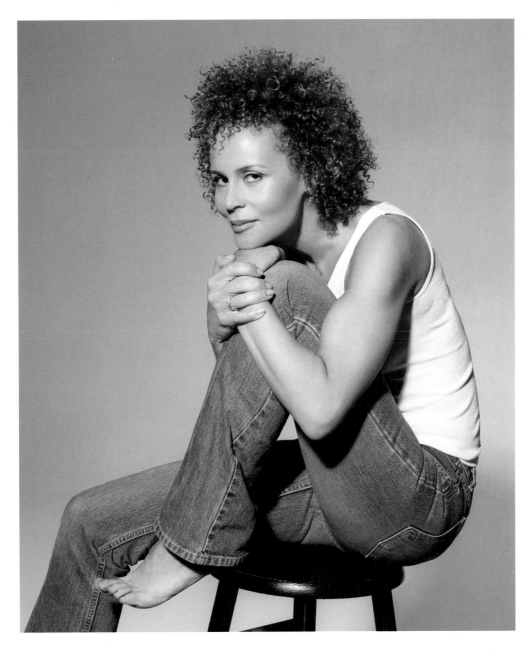

Then there are those attitudes that strengthen and tone your emotional beauty. "When it comes to my inner beauty, I'm trying to honor myself and my needs, something that has progressed with age," says actress Vanessa Williams. "When you're first starting out in your teens or twenties, you're always trying to please others, which was my case. When I reached my thirties I became much more vocal about my boundaries and honoring what my true feelings were. That was very liberating and gave me a sense of calm, which reverts back to what I think being beautiful is. It's something I struggle with but also embrace as I grow older—being true to myself," concludes Williams. And yet the truth is, despite what we put into our lives to secure them, there are curves. Williams has her own coping skills. "I have to take every moment and every period of time as it comes

*Fashion buyer
and store manager
Jennifer Thread
McHenry*

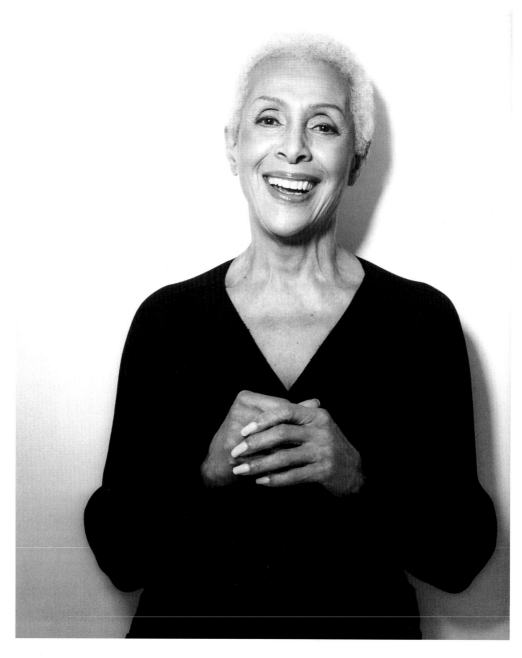

*Holistic counselor
and education specialist
Jacqueline Peters Canon*

instead of getting overwhelmed and resentful and thinking that it's going to be the same way all the time, because life changes constantly," she says. "So much of one's inner or emotional beauty has to do with the kind of thoughts you allow to move in and the kind of thoughts you're happy to say goodbye to," says Jacqueline Peters Canon, who makes it a practice to detox mentally by pushing the release button on negative thoughts first and then "letting them go!"

Honoring all that you are is key as is doing those things that affirm your core. Singer Patti LaBelle makes a point of doing those things that feed her inner and outer beauty with a purpose. "Even inside the house, I'm going to be cute! I want to see myself looking good. Beauty is in the eye of the beholder! When you catch me at a bad space in my day, I'll say okay and give myself a *Patti* day. A whole day of not worrying about if you have on a hat because it's cold outside, not worrying about if you ate, if you have on boots in the snow. Because I have these wide shoulders and it seems like everybody's problem is my burden and that's the way I am, and so I take Patti days now where I do nothing but pamper *me*. Some days I just cook for me and I say, 'I'm not including anybody in this pot.' So it's about putting myself first, and that's what a lot women have to start doing."

Establish a Temple Management Team

If you're like most sisters, you're busy seeing to everyone, from family and friends to neighbors and those simply in need—often at your own expense. Have you ever stopped to consider who's taking care of you? Have you chosen life's best support systems to maintain your temple? Is your inner and outer beauty tended, pampered, and fortified for the journey? Among the most important things I've come to value as a woman and as an editor are expert advice and support. I have become so much more just from the guidance of many experts, in both my personal and professional lives. And so I consider it essential that every woman have what I've come to call a *temple management team*—in other words, a coterie of experts that help you get and keep it together.

For me that team consists of a group of experts who help me manage both my inner and outer beauty. High on the list are my minister and my doctors—such as the Ayurvedic naturopathic doctor I see, and (new to the team) an iridologist. Iridology is a master science that uses the patterns of your eye's iris to reveal the condition of your body. These patterns develop from birth and are affected by your lifestyle and diet. Having an analysis, where an iridologist examines both the iris as well as the sclera (the whites) of the eyes by looking into them with the aid of a flashlight or by photographing them with a machine designed specifically for this purpose, is a wonderful way to determine the quality of your health, what organs are in need of repair and those that are in the process of healing, as well as determine deficiencies and establish preventive measures. More specifically, clients walk away from these exams knowing which foods, supplements, and forms of exercise will speed up the healing in a particular area.

Then there's my outer beauty team, among whom my hairstylist is chief, along with the aestheticians who help me keep the glowing skin that I love, my manicurist, and a number of experts at spas across the nation whom I see on an as-wanted-and-highly-desired basis!

For some of the women I've talked to on the journey the list is different. There are women who consult a lifestyle coach as part of their overall team to help them achieve their desires in the most practical ways that they can implement and from which they can begin to see immediate results. Some, like McHenry, rely on a personal trainer—"there are times when my trainer will fax a program for me to the hotel when I'm traveling," she says. There are those for whom a herbalist is key as they seek to manage their health from a natural perspective. Others seek counsel to help them manage a stressful life and achieve the necessary centering required to rule over it. The concept of having such a team has touched the lives of wise women of all ages. For Halle, it's her personal trainer of twelve years, Robert White; her holistic doctor; and the creative people who help her express her beauty and style. For model and actress Veronica Webb, being in control of her health—both mental and physical—allows her to control her looks. To help her achieve this control, she turns to "Kacy Duke, my personal trainer, nutritionist Oz Garcia (both of New York's Equinox Gyms), my pastor, and my psychiatrist—not necessarily in that order, though!" Webb exclaims. "And hairstylist Oscar James and makeup artist Sam Fine are the deacons in the temple!" she adds. Seriously, though, supporting your inner and outer beauty through the guidance and care of the best experts is something you should be doing for yourself without question. The rewards to your body, mind, and spirit are far too wonderful for you to miss. Think of it as a supreme form of care that you're more than deserving of. Begin to examine your needs and desires and then put the appropriate experts into place in your life to help you be all that you can be.

Take Your Cues from the Right Sources

Whom do you have confidence in? Do you have strong, supportive relationships that promote your growth? Who's got your back? Do you have a prayer partner? Strong women move through life with a support system, a crucial network of several sister friends, for they know that when it comes to the subject of their emotional beauty, they have to be careful whom they take their cues from. Here is a checklist of those sisters I think every woman should have in her coterie:

- A mentor, the woman you aspire to be like, whom you turn to for guidance with all the big questions in your life. She won't always say what you want to hear, but listen up!

- Your mom-away-from-mom—this is the sister who loves you for all that the world may not readily see, the one who's just as quick to bring you a cup of homemade soup as she is to remind you that God isn't finished with you yet, so why are you so down on the story when things don't go your way? Take her lessons in wisdom and patience and thrive!

- A no-nonsense sister friend, the one who gives you the kind of tough love that pushes you out of your pity party and into action with a prayer for whatever it is that you need to be doing. She's the one who tells you you're just the girl to make it happen, so get over it or out from under it and get to work!

- The young urbanite—this is the friend who keeps you current, who also helps you laugh at yourself and in the process stop being the star of your own dramas in life. And if you're a mother to a young teen, this is the sister who can help you understand what your daughter may be going through and how to address it—not by trying to become her friend, but by being a mother who can relate and yet not relax. You know, girls don't suddenly turn into brats any more than we suddenly turn into tyrants in their eyes; experts say it is cultivated through the process of wrong actions and wrong responses. So aside from exercising patience, listening to the clarity of a young sister friend can help.

- Finally, there's the best friend—one who's like a caring older sister who watches over you and tells you when someone or something in life is no good for you. She's the one you don't need to talk to every day but can call at 3:00 A.M. and you know she'll be right there. Furthermore, you can trust that your confidences will remain her confidences.

I have every one of the above in my life, and I can tell you I am much better for it. Like Halle, I grew up with a strong mother who taught me everything I needed for the journey ahead. She was my strongest advocate, something so significant when you're finding and ultimately maintaining your way in life. Now that she's no longer present, it's that foundation, along with the loving guidance of my sister and others, that keeps me on course. Along these lines, I've also learned to be a better friend to myself, like model Karen Alexander, whose confident beauty appears on the cover of this book, and to stop doing to myself the things I wouldn't welcome from a friend, such as negative dialogue, unconstructive criticism, and the kinds of thoughts that, as Karen says, "chip away at your character." Susan L. Taylor, whose book *Lessons in Living* guides us into the most edifying truths, reminds us that "we must all work at developing a warm friendly union and loving relationship with ourselves. We should strive to become our own best friend. Unconditional self-love and acceptance, forgiving ourselves for not taking the best care of us will free us from the deadly cycle of neglect and self-sacrifice. Our body responds to the blessings of love, praise, and gratitude; we become radiant, and splendor awakens in our heart."

Self-Edit!

What's holding you back from living the life you want? What beauty challenges do you face? How are you addressing them? The best course of action is to first open up and believe that what you desire is possible, and then plot the course that will help you to realize it. "Think about some things that are plausible, that could be attained if you work at it. If you really open up to what's possible in front of you, there are some incredible things that you may have ignored," says JoAnn Magdoff, Ph.D., a psychotherapist with a private practice in New York City. If you desire something passionately enough, "don't sell yourself short—explore it and do your research. If you really want to have muscles like someone you admire, how did they obtain them? How do you get to what you want? Really sit down and prag-matically define it. And if you hate what you're doing, think about two things: what got you there and what's keeping you there," she adds.

"When you view your life as limited, you limit your life. You don't see that grand sweep of possibilities for healing, prosperity, and peace. Simply put: What-ever you give your love, time and attention to, you get more of," says Taylor.

I have long been taught that to know better is to do better, so as I travel through life, I'm constantly editing, incorporating practices that affirm who I am and, more importantly, move me closer to my best self, whether it's exercises that strengthen my body or a class that helps me deal with conflict management. This is why I'm constantly on the lookout for experts who support both my inner and outer beauty and why I'm always checking out products and practices that not only enhance my outer beauty but in the process give me some valuable time with myself—as you'll see in the chapter that follows, time for self is crucial to total well-being and a fulfilled life. I believe looking good and feeling fabulous go hand in hand, so all my efforts focus on both. I wouldn't come in from a long day at work and go to bed with my makeup on any more than I would consume diet beverages, knowing the adverse impact such practices can have on my inner and outer beauty. Nor would I continue to surround myself with negative people or fail to fuel my vessel with the healthiest foods—moves like these would compro-mise everything I stand for, not to mention hinder me in the journey. Self-editing also includes simplifying your life so that whatever lies within your control is a snap. Certainly an elaborate makeup routine or a hairstyle that's difficult to achieve and requires constant checking is best edited out of your life—why bother when there are so many fabulous alternatives that are easy to come by and in the process edify you about who you are? For that matter, anything overly complicated should be left out of your regimen, as these are the things that'll keep you from moving through life with full assurance. In their place should be practices that you know without a doubt work for you and keep you looking fine and feeling your best!

Don't Let Adversity Stump You—Stand Firm!

How confident are you? What are you sure of? What firm commitments do you live by? In the New Testament there is a parable that talks about a house built on sandy ground. In the face of a serious storm the house fell, and the resulting damage was immense. It is contrasted with a house built on a firm foundation, which was able to withstand the floods and fierce winds.

Truth be told, in the journey that is life, every day is not Sunday, and for sure there are those times when we're all challenged, misunderstood, or nearly thrown off course. These are the times when we need to be able to stand firm, on a solid foundation, and not give in, give up, or give out! To me, this is the true meaning of endurance, for it is where preparation meets opportunity, allowing you to withstand whatever comes your way. I've learned that if you let adversity arrest you, it will surely make you its prisoner. What's key for me is not letting those ill winds toss me about, but rather using them to accelerate my spiritual growth. In fact, I find that it is in the face of challenge that I grow the most. You know that old principle about how building muscle requires that you lift some weights? Well, it's still true. This is how confidence and endurance are stoked. "I remember that I was put here to do battle, and each time I conquer a battle I come out more brand-new and more grounded and empowered," says Halle Berry, who over the years has learned how to make adversity work to her advantage. When you leap the difficult hurdles, you land a stronger person on the other side. What's key is to recognize that victory and claim it, as opposed to turning away from it. "I'm learning—I'm practicing how to relax and work with whatever appears on my path. I'm trying not to run from anything I feel or experience, whether it's the loss of my youth, material things, a relationship, or my beloved parents, or feelings of failure, embarrassment, anger, or jealousy," says Taylor, whom I admire so for her tenacity in the face of unscripted challenge and her willingness to share with others on how to overcome and grow.

I remember when Oprah went on trial in Texas for allegedly defaming the beef industry. What we saw in the media was a watchful and determined woman willing to stand behind the fact that she had done nothing wrong. What you did not see while Winfrey was on the witness stand was her ever-growing faith in the truth of who she is and the fact that no one was going to define Oprah but *her*. For Winfrey, that in and of itself was a victory, long before the trial ended with a verdict in her favor. "And that's how you find out who you really are—you've got to get quiet enough to know," something she did in the midst of the fiery trial. "You become what you believe, and if you believe somewhere, even in the most subconscious, 'I can't get this far,' that will be the thing that holds you back," Winfrey concludes.

So be determined that you won't let anything or anyone throw you off course. Make no provisions within for self-doubt, but rather, affirm yourself by focusing on all that's wonderful and true about you. Metaphorically speaking, don't leave home without your armor of faith and your shield of self-appreciation. When you get right down to it, these are the attributes that will help you stand firm.

Here's to Life!

The time has come for us to love ourselves in the highest order—to own our lives and celebrate our beauty to the fullest! We owe it to ourselves to live abundant in spirit, joyful in hope, and steady during the course of challenge. To incorporate into our lives the experiences that nourish us, and particularly those that strengthen us in the face of adversity. To learn to say no to some things that keep us busy, so we can fully say yes to those that'll move us forward, closer to fulfillment. "To go beyond, and not fall into a pattern that has been there before and grow therein," as actress LaTanya Richardson Jackson says, "but to really grow into a space that *we* have created!" And most of all, to dare to dream and then step out in faith to confirm those dreams by doing whatever it takes to make them our reality. "We should ask ourselves, 'What is my vision? Where do I want to be in my life this time next year? Five years from now? And how do I want to live my elder years?' We have to do whatever it takes to get the roadblocks and conflicts out of the way—and these can be negative people, a negative attitude, or unhealthy habits. But God is so good because each of us, no matter where we are in life at the moment, has the power to choose something better, richer, and more fulfilling for herself," says Taylor.

For the sister who established a foundation in her name to support the inspiration, empowerment, and education of women, children, and families around the world, the concept of living from within is focused and real. "When you recognize that you didn't just come to the planet to do all the little things that you do, but that you are all that the Creator intended for you to be right now—don't be afraid of it. I used to be afraid to say, 'I am Oprah Winfrey and I am all that.' I used to be afraid to own that. But what I did when I came into my forties, I gave up all the stuff: stopped reading press releases, stopped reading tabloids, stopped listening to the radio, gave up looking at the ratings—just really stopped. I said it doesn't matter, because I recognize that the things that I have

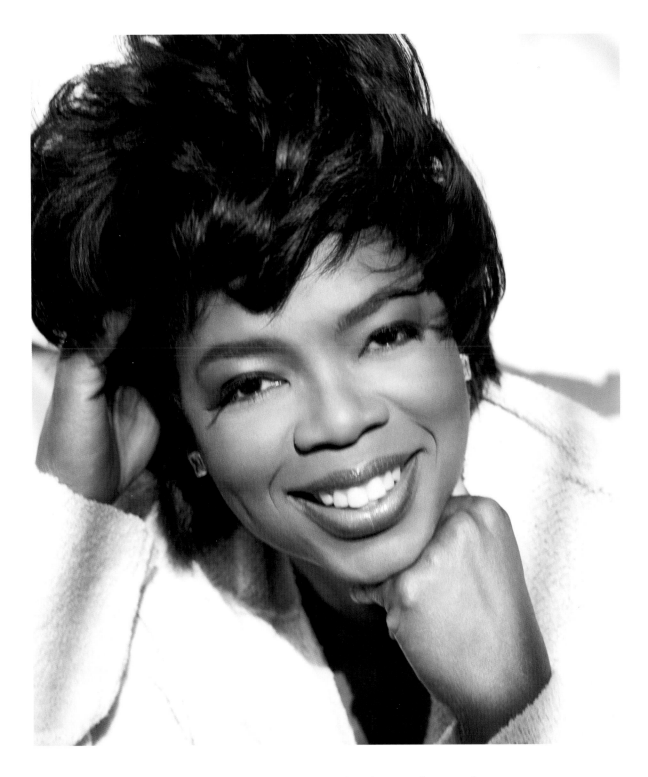

going for myself comes from a deeper, stronger, wider place, and my goal every day is to try to tap into that!" Winfrey concludes.

When all is said and done, only you can and should define what works for you in life—I'm just offering you the options. Take them and thrive. Here's to living the life you want!

Amen.

2 TIME FOR SELF

"To every thing there is a season, and a time to every purpose . . ."

ECCLESIASTES 3:1, OLD TESTAMENT

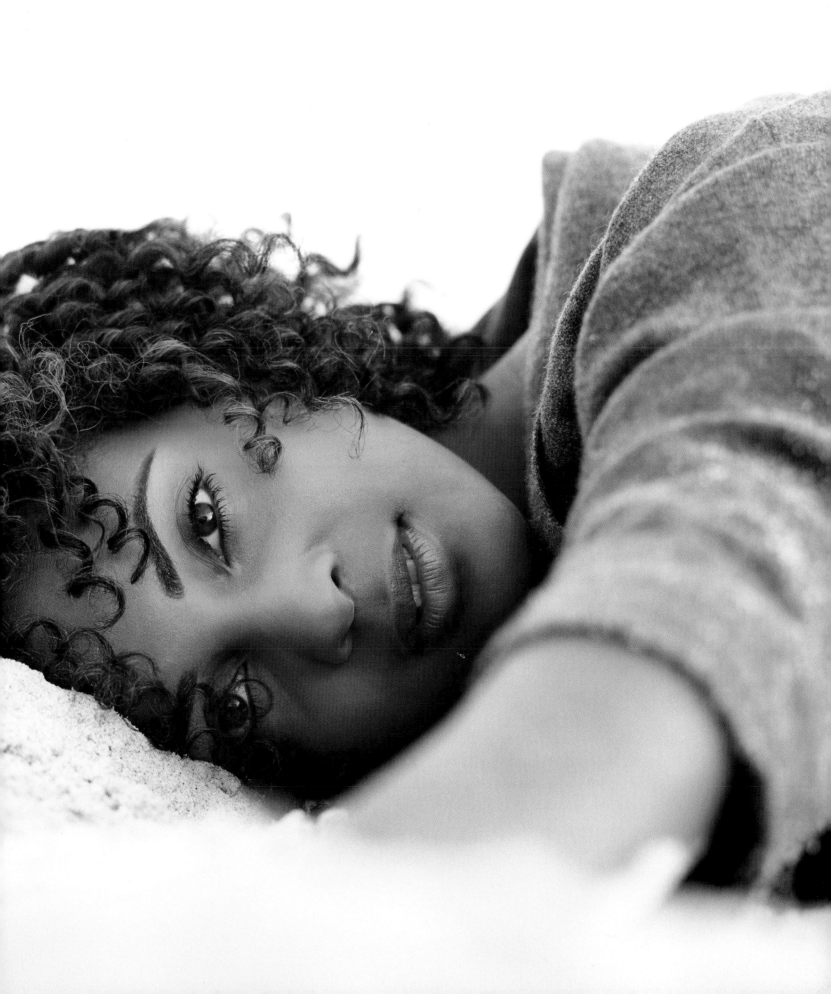

It's easy to lose sight of yourself and what's important in the busy-ness of life. I know this firsthand. I can remember a time when I used to hit the ground running with a mental to-do list that had far more entries than even two people could accomplish in one day! It was a time when my body, mind, and spirit occupied different places, and I thought I was sister "every woman."

I can clearly recall what those seventeen-hour days of storming from one thing to the next and pushing my body like a machine were like, because it's a state of being that I never want to know again. I ran mostly on empty during that time, trying to serve everyone and everything as if my tank were full. My poor mind couldn't absorb the peace of sleep; it just kept on working long after my body had shut down. As for tending to my physical beauty, it was solely about keeping up an appearance, meaning put the makeup on and get the hair done! Needless to say, I often took myself for granted and placed my name at the bottom of my priority list under "good intentions." I seldom got that far down the list because I kept running out of time and energy, and I didn't realize the importance of it. But let me tell you, sisters, this is a path that will wear out your body, destroy your good looks, and cripple your mind and spirit quicker than anything, because it's not only stressful, it's neglectful! We are supreme beings and we need to set aside time to nurture and restore ourselves daily—that's part of how we give evi-dence that *we* know how special we are. So I've learned that despite how many people we belong to or are responsible for, before we can effectively move in their worlds, we need to move in ours! JoAnn Magdoff, Ph.D., a psychotherapist in New

York City, reminds us, "You have to make time for yourself, otherwise you can't really take on any of your other responsibilities with an open heart!" Part of being effective is learning to say no to some things, and that's difficult for many of us to do simply because we hate to disappoint others, especially those we love. This often leads to taking on more than we can reasonably handle. It also means working in a cooperative spirit with ourselves, agreeing to listen to what's going on inside us so that we don't overtax ourselves. It's important to be discerning and give what I've come to call a reasonable order to our days by learning to strike a balance. Fran Sachs, a mind-body fitness therapist at Manhattan's Sea Change Healing Center, told me that we need to adopt the attitude that "what I did today was enough." A wise sister friend called me up one day to remind me that God is not scattered, He's focused! So whenever you think that you've come up short, remember that even God rested from calling creation into existence.

We also need to learn to step away purposefully from the busyness of everyday life. Notice I didn't say "steal away" or "sneak off," common expressions we use when we go to take care of ourselves. Step away—you're in charge! And don't be afraid or ashamed to do so. Learn to be comfortable about placing yourself at the top of your priority list and scheduling some time for self every day. Sheryl Lee Ralph, star of the former hit TV series *Moesha*, admits sometimes it's not bad to be a little self-centered. "You know that expression 'Take care of home first'? Well, you have to take care of self first," says Ralph, who takes her quiet time whenever the need arises and does "absolutely nothing!" She points out that it's really about knowing when to stop and be kind to yourself.

Now that I've got the lesson, I rise every morning about an hour before my family and use that quiet time to meditate, pray, and then tend to my body. I also give myself the gift of some additional time at the end of the day to tune the world out and turn inward. Come Sunday, I'll use this precious hour of solitude to restore body, mind, and spirit through an exfoliating body scrub, followed by a de-stressing bath coupled with an affirming read. I usually enhance this experience with the healing sound of an environmental CD or classical music and a soothing cup of herbal tea. I also schedule some time each month to be pampered and tended to in ways that allow me to thoroughly let go. For example, I love the experience of having a professional pedicure, so I make sure that I schedule time to kick back and have one about every four weeks. I also block out time for facials and massages as often as I can. The benefits of these treatments go much farther than the eye can see, for they not only give me a much-needed break and a beautifying treat but are special gifts of time that allow for some personal reflection while rejuvenating my mind and my spirit in the process. These escapes represent just a few of the many ways that I routinely make time for myself.

Since I've come to know the importance of it, I'm always on the lookout for ways, great and small, to step away and have some quiet time of restoration.

Each of us has some time that we can devote to ourselves, whether at the start or the close of the day or smack dab in the middle—which might mean taking a rejuvenating lunch break in the beautiful solitude of a nearby park. My friend Bonnie McDaniel, author of *In the Eye of the Storm*, loves to garden. She steps away each day for the restoring process of "working the good earth," as she puts it. While it may appear to her neighbors that she's simply tending her garden, McDaniel is in fact tending her sacred space—her mind. It has been a ritual of hers ever since I've known her, and it works. Star Jones, a cohost of ABC's *The View* (who made a point of telling me that she's very comfortable with her own silence), routinely turns her phone off for a period every day. Says Star, "If you don't take that time, people will really and truly take advantage of you!" From her perspective, the phone is for her convenience, so for a short time each afternoon she turns it off, lights a candle, and enjoys a quiet, meditative repose. For actress Vanessa Williams, it's that lovely slice of time in the shower where she gains an essential calm with the use of scented shower gels. She also escapes to the sea, which she says "clears my mind and makes me feel grounded." The point, my sisters, is this: The main event here is you, and all I'm saying is to give some serious thought to what works for you and direct your life from there. It's a plan that will pay off, both now and for years to come. It will also inspire those around you to follow suit. While we may not realize it, the attitudes that our daughters and younger sisters often take on are directly influenced by the way they see us regard ourselves. I can't tell you how much of an effort I've made to make sure my children don't see me as someone who's overloaded and always in a hurry. That's not the message I want them to take away—nor do I want it to be my truth. So know that it's important not only to nurture ourselves in this way but to set an example that will inform others with the right thinking as well.

This quality time with ourselves is not an option or a luxury—and it certainly isn't anything to feel guilty about. It is an essential form of self-renewal. We are body, mind, and spirit, and we need to make time daily to connect and tend all three. This is what self-renewal is all about. It begins at the center, with your mind. Scripture says in Proverbs 4:23: "Keep thy heart with all diligence; for out of it are the issues of life." As I've noted, the term *heart* is used in the Bible to refer to the mind. The directive is this: Tend or guard your mind with meticulous care, for it is the center from which your every action is directed.

The chamber of your mind is your "command central," the place where all of your thoughts are conceived. Like an air traffic controller, you have the power to direct these thoughts, and ultimately your actions, in the direction you want them to go. Therefore, it is so important to do some housekeeping in your mind, so to speak, in order that you might reflect and make sure that the kinds of directives and information that are dwelling there are useful to your body and your spirit.

Equally important, your mind is the place where peace is realized and where you have a deep communion with God and yourself. Herein lies your wealth, so don't fail to make a daily investment. This is where knowledge meets power. It's how you gain and keep clarity, focus, direction, and a beauty that is rich beyond measure. Personally, I could not live without this loving and reflective time alone with myself and with my Creator, for this is a source of renewal for me and a proven measure for staying balanced. Beauty experts say that the mind is a storehouse of power, more capable of producing the radiance that we seek than anything in a bottle or a jar. When you think about it, this is no mystery. Take, for example, the look of a woman in love. She's radiant! Why? Because her mind is being tended with love, time, and devotion! The radiance that is evident upon her face is really the outward effects of her inner feelings—it is clearly a case of mind over matter—and it is real. According to *ESSENCE* columnist and psychologist Gwendolyn Goldsby Grant, Ed.D., of Newark, New Jersey, what you think in your mind and the way you feel reflects itself in your skin, your eyes, and how you walk through the world. So spending time tending your mind is an empowering action that's beneficial not only to your inner beauty but to your outer beauty as well.

Self-renewal requires that you be grandiose in appraising your total well-being. It causes you to stay focused and to realize that body, mind, and spirit need to operate in accord. Just as scripture makes reference to our minds, it also speaks about our bodies. The New Testament refers to our bodies as temples, and if you relate this to earthen temples, you know that they are beautiful, sacred places that are always well tended. We must care for ourselves with the same regard and focus on every aspect of our being. Likewise, we must tend our spirits, like our bodies and our minds; they too need exercise, tuning, and a period for restoration. And you have to give order to the power that lies within you to make this happen on a daily basis. Otherwise you'll find yourself in a battle for both your inner and your outer beauty, for when your body, mind, and spirit are disconnected, so are you! Clearly this is yet another reason why spending time with yourself is so important. How can you give order to what you have set as a purpose for yourself if you don't come away from the busyness of life to focus on it and seek wisdom and direction? Use this time and vital form of communication to recognize who you are, how you're doing and moving through life. Far too many sisters say they feel out of touch with themselves and don't even know where the time goes. When you are in touch, you always know what time it is in your life—and that's enough! This vital aspect of self-seduction is crucial to your being whole, for it is a nurturing experience that will keep your inner and outer beauty in the flow. It will also keep you anchored in a state of grace, an outstanding characteristic of any beautiful woman. Actress Phylicia Rashad, who's known as much for her regal personality as she is for her striking good looks, says she maintains her calm and graciousness through meditation. Rashad, who rises every day before dawn to meditate for fifteen minutes to an hour, says, "It's like keeping a sacred place clean." She uses this practice to focus her mind, examine the quality of her thinking, and release any negativity. The actress says she finds her center there and it remains with her throughout the day—"no matter what is going on," she adds! Ditto for Oprah Winfrey, who declares that without this affirming practice, her day becomes disarrayed and she just can't pull it back together. Winfrey, who commits to this daily time with herself, also uses this time to order her spirit with the mantra "I am that which comes from God." "You say that to yourself for just a minute and you understand the depth and power of that and it just puts everything in its place," she says, and adds that this allows her to know that there's a bigger reason for whatever it is she's about to do. I laughed when she told me how this takes the emphasis off the stuff that can unravel us, such as *I can't find my shoes, where's my keys* et cetera. I've sweated the small stuff enough to know just what she's talking about! Know too that experts concur that starting your day off in the quiet of your own company with positive affirmations is a good practice. "When you wake up, visualize the world you want for today," says Grant, and she adds, "As you're creating new thoughts for the day ahead, this is a perfect time to say, 'Out with the old and in with the new!'" Far too many times, our mental bags are so overloaded with the concerns of yesterday that it's a wonder we can move forward to accept the opportunities a new day brings. But don't let this be true of you— commit to leaving the past in the past, and accept each day with gratitude.

Truth be told, oftentimes our little beauty frustrations, such as ill tempers, bad moods, lack of direction, and what I call physical chaos, stem from this simple omission: failing to take time to nurture ourselves. These negatives give evidence that we've lost our connection to self, and there's nothing beautiful about that. Given the power that lies at our fingertips, this should never be. So I say put your wish list away and stop hoping that one day you'll have time to relax, clear your mind, and be good to yourself. Instead, reorder your steps so that you turn inward some of the love you lavish on others. Know that it's easier than you think, for there's a healing fountain that lies within each of us and various methods by which to draw from it. And trust me—once you start carving out your special time, you'll not only incorporate many of the following practices, you'll get creative and add to the list!

Meditate

In its simplest form, meditation is a devotional exercise of contemplation; more deeply, it is a cultivation of the spirit. Both forms have been practiced by our ancestors for hundreds of years. In Africa, many of the elders, priests, kings, and queens used this powerful technique to hone their mental skills in order to effectively lead and guide our people. Ra Un Nefer Amen, author of several books, including *The Tree of Life Meditation System*, says, "The ancestors understood that there were two parts of us and of course the inner part was the greater and more powerful—it determined the external aspects of our lives."

According to Queen Afua, of the Heal Thyself Natural Living Center in Brooklyn, New York, they also used meditation to unleash their spirituality. "Our ancestors looked at the body not only in the physical sense, but also as spiritual," she states. They believed meditation linked them to the Creator, and they even wore meditative symbols on their crowns.

Today, on the path to beauty and wellness, meditation is a compass that continually guides us onto higher ground by causing us to be still and pay attention to ourselves. I am amazed sometimes when I think about how many people we as women can belong to at any given time in our lives! When you couple that with juggling the pressures of life, unforeseen responsibilities, and seemingly endless to-do lists, it's no wonder many of us feel like "arrival time" isn't what we thought it would be—because we never have any time for ourselves. Truth is, you have to make time for yourself and label it a priority. Susan L. Taylor, editorial director of *ESSENCE* magazine, puts it this way: "You have to give yourself to yourself before you give yourself away." Turning inward through the practice of meditation is one of several richly rewarding ways to do so. Actress Halle Berry routinely carves out time alone in her daily schedule to nurture herself in this way. "I'm finding that it's really important so I can hear my own voice," she states. Berry says she's in a business where so many people are telling her what to do that it's important to take the time to hear what her intuition is telling her, and so she meditates daily, anywhere from forty-five minutes to an hour or more when time permits.

According to the experts, meditation should be a way of life given the fast pace of most of our lives because it reduces stress, increases energy, and awakens our intuition. Moreover, it allows us to shut down the awareness of what's going on around us and focus inward to a quieter and deeper level of ourselves. Examining our lives from the inside out is one of the many ways in which we can open up and come face-to-face with that healing fountain I spoke of earlier. Sometimes it's simply a matter of asking ourselves, "How are you doing?" and then responding on every level and shaping our perspective and plans accordingly. This in and of itself is both cleansing and healing, as it gives us the information we need to put and keep our lives in order. Other times it's a matter of rejuvenating mind, body, and spirit through meditative visualization, a sort of self-guided imagery in which you imagine yourself in a tranquil setting, such as on a beautiful beach. This form of meditation can alter your subconscious and immediately help you to relax. In addition, research has shown that calming the mind can help quell headaches, insomnia, and other stressful conditions such as PMS. Furthermore, experts at Harvard University–affiliated hospitals and clinics have concluded that spending ten minutes a day in meditation can reduce your heart rate and blood pressure as well as significantly slow secretions of the stress hormone cortisol, which has been linked to weight gain.

One of the great benefits of meditation is that it is so easy to do. You can practice it in the privacy of your home, in your office, or in a setting that puts you in tune with nature, such as an open field; Halle sometimes meditates while sitting out in the rain. You can even get creative and devise your own sacred space expressly for this purpose, like actress Loretta Devine did by converting a small, closetlike space in her house—a very purposeful way to invoke this practice and invite transformation. I meditate in a number of spaces within my bedroom and bathroom. These are the rooms where I close the door on the world and step into my private space, so they represent the perfect setting for me. My friend Betty Barkley, a claims adjuster for a nationwide insurance agency, meditates on her evening walk. Some elder sisters, like my grandmother and yours, used to meditate while rocking in a chair. Wherever and however you choose to journey within, remember this: Concentration and mindful breathing are key to guarantee retreat and renewal.

Begin right now to enjoy the fruits of meditation by setting aside a special time for it. Be consistent and stay committed so that you can reach your full potential and the practice becomes effortless. Remember, any form of introspection is a valuable opportunity for renewal. With meditation, the rewards are extraordinary.

Here's a simple way to start:

- Choose a place where you can be quiet for ten to fifteen minutes. If you're at your desk, turn off your computer and let your calls go into voicemail.

- Get comfortable—sit on the floor or in a chair in an upright position, shoulders down and your back as straight as possible.

- Close your eyes and let go—release all thoughts of the outside world and any pent-up tension. Consciously step within.

- Begin to be aware of your breathing. Take a long deep breath in and then slowly blow it out, consciously relaxing as you do so.

- Continue to focus on your breathing and the quality of your thinking. If distracting thoughts try to invade, simply acknowledge their presence, let go, and return to your focus.

- When you're ready to conclude, return to your normal breathing pattern. Sit quietly for a few moments and then open your eyes.

- Take a few minutes to record your thoughts, revelations, and any course of action you need to take.

Once you've become comfortable with this practice, begin to turn inward more deeply and examine yourself and the life you are living. Learn to listen to your inner voice, empty any negativity dwelling in your consciousness, and affirm your desires. Enrich your life further by setting aside time to just center on the Divine by taking the Word into meditation. Scripture says in Isaiah 26:3, "Thou wilt keep him in perfect peace, whose mind is stayed on thee." Needless to say, peace is something we all savor in this day and age; scripture offers us this insight as to how it can be maintained. By meditating on the Word, we also gain clarity concerning our true value in life, and if we use this knowledge assertively, we ultimately get closer to God and begin to live out the empowered life He desires for us. According to Psalms 104:34, it will also keep you on higher ground in the day-to-day by sweetening your outlook.

To help you relish this time for self, you might enhance it further with a scented candle or incense, or by adding essential oils to a lamp ring. If you choose to meditate in the bath, a ceremony I find very conducive to introspection, add a few drops of an essential oil such as lemon, which is uplifting, to your water. According to the folks at Aura Cacia, a leading manufacturer of pure essential oils, aromatherapy and meditation work together—essential oils work like a key to unlock our sensory system triggering memory and emotions in the limbic system of the brain. When stimulated, the limbic system releases chemicals that affect our central nervous system, counteracting adverse feelings such as anxiety, pain, and negativity. Used to complement a meditative state, aromatherapy can help you achieve a balanced, insightful frame of mind.

You can also enhance the practice of meditation by the foods you eat. "There are calming foods and agitative foods," says Queen Afua. She cites greens such as watercress and wheatgrass and beverages such as cucumber juice and alfalfa tea as having the ability to open up the psyche and allow you to be in a state of meditation. She includes fruits and vegetables as pluses too, as they help to rejuvenate and purify your temple, both of which play a role in effective meditation. Afua reminds us that the purpose of meditation is to charge the spirit, and advocates that we steer clear of sugar, which she says agitates and depletes the spirit.

Pray

In our quest to enrich and beautify, prayer is one spirit-nourishing tool that we should invoke daily. Through divine communication we are clarified, renewed, and empowered to be our higher selves. "The ability to sit down and to pray is cleansing," says Star Jones of ABC's *The View*, who'll tell you in no uncertain terms about the value of being able to ask God to order your steps. "Life can hand you some pretty ugly things," she says, "but if you just say, 'Lord, direct me,' you can rise above it all." I know personally it is this support system that keeps my emotional well-being in the flow. What I find unfortunate in our fast-moving times is how prayer has come to represent a formulaic speech before meals or a plea when we're in distress. Model Karen Alexander told me she could relate to this, as one day she realized that she had to stop the deal-making prayers that she offered to God. Instead, she began to really talk to Him and give Him the proper place in her life. Now this busy model and mother of two says she stays in a constant state of prayer, as she finds guidance and confirmation therein. Karen's not alone in this self-examination; quite frankly I too remember those times when I myself was guilty of sending God a number of e-mails posing as prayer! But to learn better is to do better, and today my life is much richer because I've come to realize that prayer is really a healing conversation with God, whose beautifying wisdom and power are available 24/7. Through prayer I'm able to release my burdens, send up my hopes, and give thanks for a joy that the stressors of life cannot quench. So when you step away to take your quiet time— whether to reflect or plan or simply because you're in need of rejuvenation— I encourage you to consider making prayer a part of the process.

Strive for Graciousness

It has been said that beauty is as beauty does. To me graciousness signals whether your beauty is about physical practices or whether it abides deep within. It is a profound awareness that is reflected not only in the way you treat others but also in the kindness you extend to yourself. Harriette Cole, author of *How to Be*, a practical guide on the fundamentals of everyday living, told me a few years ago that we have to pay attention to our presentation both on the inside and on the outside. Cole cites this focus as one way to avoid falling into the trap she refers to as "How do I look?" She's right. True beauty is more substantive than that; it's about conscious living from within. When we are calm and collected, there's an order to our world and we're able to move mind over matter and keep our perspective. We are in sync with ourselves and are easily able to treat others the way we wish to be treated. How we nurture ourselves through self-affirming rituals has a lot to do with it. According to San Francisco family psychologist Dr. Brenda Wade, we must be committed to taking the time to honor our body temple as well as to speaking words of encouragement and love to ourselves in our inner dialogue. Wade encourages us to chant over and over in our minds—and out loud when we can—such affirmations as "I am worthy, I am an enlightened person, I am an uplifting person, I am a success." Simply put: If we want to be gracious, we must affirm this attribute within first. Ultimately it will be the gift that we give to others.

How connected we are to the Creator also plays a role in how gracious we are. This relationship can infuse us with a peace that takes the edge off life's pressures and anchors us in a true state of graciousness. Being rooted in this realm is what will enable us to go the distance. It will also cause us to "esteem one another highly," as the scripture says, and commit acts of kindness that make the world a prettier place because we're in it.

When you strive for graciousness, there are certain practices that you won't allow to be true about you, such as gossiping about others, being overly critical, backbiting, and envious of another's success. Characteristics like these spoil your beauty and hinder your growth. They also cause you to overlook the gifts and opportunities the Creator has uniquely given you by distracting you with the concerns and successes of others. Aim, then, to resist these negative tendencies at all costs and replace them with positive practices that lift you and all of us in the process. Habits of a truly gracious woman include:

■ She's swift to hear, slow to speak, and slow to anger (James 1:19 New Testament).

■ She's patient.

■ She's known for her impeccable manners; the mainstays of "please" and "thank you" are always a part of her conversation.

■ She always reaches out to others and is known to give more than she ever takes.

■ She knows how to bond and keep relationships.

■ She honors those secrets that have been entrusted to her.

Think of graciousness as a way of staying in touch with the beauty within you and those who came before you. Recognize that you represent kings, queens, priests, priestesses, and survivors of the Maafa—even your immediate ancestors, who have known many a sacrifice with great dignity that you might possess the life that you now know. In representing your rich heritage, do so with honor, courtesy, kindness, poise, and a queenly dignity that tells the world you know who you are and what you possess. Know, as singer Nancy Wilson so eloquently put it to me when I asked her about her own graciousness, that "this is your God-ness, the evidence that you're special and He loves you!"

Catch Your Breath!

Today, more often than not, given our modern-day attitudes and self-imposed pace in life, many of us are waiting to inhale. We are in such a hurry to say more, do more, be more, that we don't realize that we are just breathing to live—taking what I call those short survival breaths in our upper chest, as opposed to breathing deeply in our lower abdomen to give our body all that it needs. We don't quite realize that proper breathing refuels our bodies and calms and relaxes us by making us focus and slow down. Nor do we know just how crucial it is to our well-being. Talk about neglecting time for self—why, we don't even take the time to breathe nowadays! But the truth is, those quickie breaths that many of us get by on, which merely bring in oxygen and take out carbon dioxide, are no way to live when compared to the deep healing breaths that center us and shore up our wellness. This hasty, improper breathing not only does our bodies a disservice but, according to the experts, has been linked to a lack of energy and a low resistance to illness, and has been cited as a reason why some of us so easily fall prey to the blues. According to Dr. Deborah G. Musso of Manhattan's Sea Change Healing Center, even such conditions as chronic fatigue syndrome have been linked to the breath. "If you're not getting enough oxygen, you will feel tired all of the time," she points out, and adds, "If you're not breathing at an optimal level, your life force is diminished, as breathing moves energy to all parts of the body." Moreover, breath has a direct link to our mind and our emotions. "When we're angry, the breath becomes tight and a little more rapid; when we're feeling relaxed, the breath slows down and becomes more rhythmic," says Krishna Kaur, who's both a yoga instructor and founding president of the International Association of Black Yoga Teachers, which is based in Los Angeles. So if we're able to control the breath and expand the mind through the breath, as Kaur suggests, we'll at least have control over our response to those things that can sometimes push our buttons. When you think about it, we grew up being told over and over again to slow down and take a deep breath. And according to Kaur, this practice still has great benefits. In the heat of an angry moment, if we just "dare to be still and take a long deep breath, exhale gently and freely, we can then take in all the elements of what's going on and respond creatively and appropriately." She adds affirmatively, "This is all controlled by the breath." How? you might ask. Kaur says that this simple practice of conscious breathing puts "one to two degrees of separation between us and the event taking place and our response to it."

Now, if you're like me, breathing is not something you think about, but that doesn't mean you're doing it properly. In fact, you might have forgotten and may need to learn anew just what it feels like. I can honestly say that despite all my learning about its importance, I still have to make a deliberate effort sometimes. We'd all like to believe that we know how to breathe; after all, we've been doing it our entire lives! But there is a proper way, and that is inhaling through the nose, filling up the lungs and engaging the diaphragm, and then exhaling through the mouth. Learning to reconnect with your breath and reap all the benefits may take some time, but like all things, practice makes perfect.

Keep a Journal

Keeping a journal teaches you a lot about yourself. It helps you get in touch with you, take your own pulse, and truly know how you're doing—down deep. It is within our journals that we can share our innermost thoughts, get a grip, reflect, make our confessions, even release our fears without criticism and gain clarity on loving and appreciating ourselves. We may carry around negatively programmed thoughts about our beauty and ultimately our lives for years without ever realizing that they exist and are holding us back from being our best selves. We also carry our unfulfilled desires around and never stop to create the plan to bring them to life. But when we sit down and begin to reflect on the clean, fresh pages of truth—which is what a journal offers—we can see clearly where we need to reassess, nourish our spirits, and go forward. In this respect, a journal becomes a blessing that calls us to grow and courageously leap onto higher heights.

Journals can also teach us a lot about the affirming power of God. Exzora Bey, one of my sisters in the spirit, told me one day to keep track in a journal of the challenges that God has brought me through. By committing to this simple practice, she said, I would have example after example of how God always brings us through—no matter what the test or trial. Today this journal is written on the pages of my heart. Now whenever I find myself facing a challenge or simply feeling overwhelmed, all I do is turn to my own record of God's favor, and believe me, it's all the encouragement I need that victory will be mine!

Without question, journals are a form of confirmation that's good for the soul. There's nothing like being able to track your own progress. It gives evidence, as celebrity makeup artist Sam Fine is quick to point out, that life is rich already—and reminds you that you're not waiting for completion, but rather adding to the story! So why not seek out the most beautiful blank book you can find, treat yourself to a lovely pen (perhaps with a shade of ink that brings you joy), and begin to share the thoughts of your heart? You can also fill it with bits of visual inspiration, such as beautiful vistas clipped from magazines, poetry, verses of scripture—whatever brings you insight and inspiration and can help you step away from the world and just spend time with you.

Take a Healing Bath

Bathing, and creatively taking it to the next level, is also another pleasurable way to reconnect with yourself. One of the best investments I ever made in my emotional well-being was to remodel my bathroom and turn it into the haven I desired. A few years ago I came to a point in my life where I decided it wasn't about jumping on a plane to find peace of mind and paying someone to pamper me, but creating a sanctuary at home to heal myself. Thanks to a little vision and one savvy carpenter, I now retreat to a lovely white-tiled space complete with adjustable lighting, music, and a sunken whirlpool bath. There, as I relax against the pulsating jets while warm fragrant water swirls around me, my healing begins. Bathing in this manner has become a purposeful ritual that cleanses and restores my body, mind, and spirit. Since I never fail to come away from this experience feeling totally renewed, I enjoy making time for it, setting out my treats and tools as they do at some of my favorite spas and then honoring myself with an ultimate soak.

To me, bathing is also a great de-stressing practice, one that's easily accessible and affordable. In fact, it's one of the least expensive escapes I can think of. Seeking solace in the private sanctuary of the bath at the end of a harried day is a welcome retreat. It allows us to put distance between ourselves and the world and to renew in solitude. Quieting the world can be easily enhanced by adding the practice of aromatherapy and color therapy, which is based on the relation between colors and our chakras. Aromatherapy seduces our senses and, when the proper ingredients are chosen, easily transports us to a state of calm and balance through the use of flowers, herbs, and plants, all of which work by sending signals to the brain. It's as easy as filling a muslin bag with rosemary, basil, dill, mint, thyme, sage, and chamomile (all of which can be grown in the kitchen) for an herbal soak that's a great sensory de-stresser. Or try adding a few

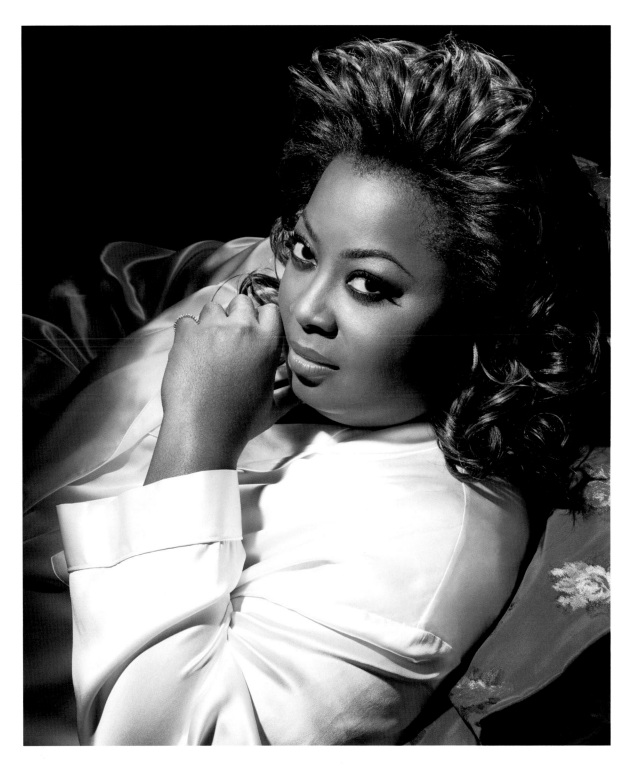

*Talk-show host
Star Jones*

drops of such essential oils as lavender and sandalwood to a warm bath in order to promote a sense of calm and peace (for additional recipes using essential oils, see "Anoint Your Body"). Even practices such as lighting a fragrant candle infused with a soothing and healing essential oil such as jasmine (as Star Jones does) or kicking back with an eye pillow filled with dried herbs designed to relax and invoke a sense of well-being are great, easily accessible de-stressers. In addition, practicing color therapy in your choice of tiles, paint, bath accessories, and bath products can also influence your mood. Experts say selecting white or paler shades of pink, violet, or green will promote harmony, spirituality, and calm. In this stressful age, tuning out the world with these concentrated efforts can make all the difference in how much disorder and tension we internalize. Our ancestors knew the value of self-nurturing rituals such as bathing, and we should recognize the same. What's key is carving out a time that you will commit to and knowing that you deserve this quiet time of renewal. For Oprah, whose days are jam-packed beyond belief, morning bubble baths have become part of her ritual to get centered before going to work. As she puts it, "Bathing for me isn't about bathing, it's about settling in with myself." She finds that this peaceful repose not only allows her to get back to herself but spurs her creativity as well. Why not schedule time for self at dawn, with a reflective soak that incorporates watching the sun rise? If you're not a morning person, step into your fountain of rejuvenation at night, after details such as returning phone calls and attending to the needs of family and friends are all taken care of. And if you really want to reward yourself, think about investing in a heated towel rack, and stack it with a big fluffy bath sheet to coddle yourself after this time of renewal. The important point to take note of is that bathing offers us more than just physical cleansing—it's a healing experience that purges body, mind, and spirit of the toxins of stress, leaving us renewed and refreshed.

Anoint Your Body

The practice of anointing dates back to biblical times. The word literally means to pour oil upon, and was an act of honoring the body as sacred. (The very thought of this will cause you to un-hurry your ways and take time for self!) You see, in ancient times, women of color tended themselves in ways that honored their bodies and their sense of self as a way of life. More often than not, in the quiet of their abodes, our foresisters went about the acts of beautifying, affirming, and ultimately appreciating their uniqueness as though they were sacred rituals. These acts of love were performed with an intensity that blessed their vessel and their mind. Central to these practices was the power of touch, a confirming action that nourishes both inner and outer beauty. From the slow and purposeful ritual of cleansing to the deliberate lubrication of their brown bodies with distinctive oils, sisters tended to their needs and desires with a unifying intention. This is who *you* are, and why it's so important for you to move beyond the basics and into the realm of conscious care—because it not only allows you to thrive but influences how you treat others. I know that when I don't take the time to consciously love and appreciate myself, I come up short with those I care about most deeply. And since I don't want this to be true of me, I've changed the way I treat myself. One of the greatest joys I now embrace in my morning ritual is that of anointing myself with aromatherapy oils that reflect my mood and my desires at the beginning of each day.

According to Mindy Green, director of education services for the Herb Research Foundation in Boulder, Colorado, "anointing brings a connotation of a state of mind that says take a minute to slow down, breathe and relax." Depending on the essential oil you use, different types of feelings are induced. "The oils create these feelings as they are absorbed through the skin or inhaled into the lungs and the brain," explains Green. Brain wave studies have shown that certain smells activate either beta waves (waves that stimulate) or alpha waves (waves that relax).

The first time I actually engaged in this practice I experienced a feeling of euphoria I'll never forget. I began by pouring a massage oil containing the essential oils of grapefruit and cypress from shoulder to shoulder, across my collarbone. I was swept away, both by the feel of the oil as it made contact with my skin and by the gesture. I realized then that this was a practice that was going to stay in my life.

Now I not only look forward to the rejuvenation anointing brings but also enjoy experiencing the many different massage oils I've accumulated to stir my desires further. Sometimes I make my own blends to achieve a specific purpose. For example, if I awake feeling sluggish, I know a blend of the essential oils of rosemary, cypress, arnica, and spearmint will stimulate my mind, aid in concentration, ease any muscle tension, and uplift my spirits. If I have a challenging day ahead, I'll try a centering blend containing lavender and cardamom or ylang-ylang and sandalwood to shore me up. I complete my ritual of solitary honor by massaging myself with both long and circular strokes all the way down to my feet. Afterward I slip into a lovely chemise, and I'm ready to move.

Learning to appreciate yourself through such acts of TLC will cause you to be an incredible woman, wife, friend, and mother. The simple act of anointing imbues you with the gifts of sensitivity and serenity, traits any beautiful woman possesses. It even gives you the proper perspective on time and allows you to see how much of it you really control. When all is said and done, it's just a question of what really takes precedence in your mind.

To this day, I can't recall hearing an elder sister use the term *routine* or *hurry* about any practice that pertained to the very personal care of her vessel. I guess that's why women like my late maternal grandmother always made time for us and those in our community—because she had an intimate, caring relationship with herself that she made time for. Her caress could still any hurt or sorrow I might have known as a child, because she knew the power of touch first-

Using essential oils to affect one's emotions is an ancient practice that has cultural origins. According to Ra Un Nefer Amen, our ancestors used a vast number of oils as inhalants, in baths, and in incense for specific purposes, among them to influence behavior. Their use was controlled by the priests, who with wisdom and understanding prescribed them to our people.

Today, essential oils are an integral part of many spa treatments, from massage and hydrotherapy baths to body wraps and facials. At home, they are the perfect transporters on the path to beauty and wholeness. To get you started, see the chart of some popular essential oils and their benefits, as well as the recipes of my favorite blends. Keep in mind that essential oils should never be applied directly to the skin, as they can cause irritation, burning, and in some cases photosensitivity. The proper way to utilize them is to dilute them with a carrier oil, such as almond, jojoba, or sesame oil. To create your own blend, use an eyedropper (which you can purchase at your local pharmacy) and add ten to twelve drops of an essential oil per ounce of carrier oil. Finally, always store your oil away from heat and light to preserve its freshness and potency.

ESSENTIAL OIL	BENEFITS
Clary sage	*Relaxing, uplifting, counters stress; aphrodisiac*
Cypress	*Sharpens mental focus, purpose; relieves fatigue and stress*
Grapefruit	*Rejuvenating; counters jet lag and the blues*
Lavender	*Relaxing, stress-relieving; reduces tension headaches*
Neroli	*Calming; quells anxiety*
Orange	*Energizing; relieves depression*
Rose	*Comforting; relieves depression, fear, stress*
Rosemary	*Improves memory; reduces fatigue and muscle tension*
Sandalwood	*Relaxing; aids in meditation; relieves insomnia; aphrodisiac*
Spearmint	*Invigorating; increases clarity, sense of well-being*
Ylang-ylang	*Antidepressant; calming; reduces anger and frustration*

Whether I'm looking to jump-start myself during a period of sluggishness or to slow down, relax, and perhaps meditate, here are some of my favorite blends to help me achieve my purpose:

Relaxation	*Lavender, sandalwood*
Energy Boosters	*Rosemary, spearmint; rosemary, grapefruit*
Concentration, Meditation	*Cypress, rosemary*
Balance	*Ylang-ylang, sandalwood*
Seduction	*Ylang-ylang, clary sage*

hand. This healing power is still a great mystery in many cases. Medical experts continue to marvel at how it works with drug-addicted babies, who might die without it. As it is essential to these struggling newborns, it is also essential to each of us. Oftentimes we overlook the power of touch even though it is at our own fingertips. This should not be. As a woman, you should appreciate the joy of your own touch and, dare I say, know your body more intimately than your significant other. Think of anointing and self-massage, then, as opportunities to fine-tune your innate sense of awareness and really get to know your entire self. Use this quiet time not only to stroke your body and ultimately your mind but also to serve a higher purpose—why not perform your monthly breast self-exam through these pleasurable rituals? It's also a good time to take inventory of your skin and any changes that might occur. While massaging myself one morning I discovered an unusual mark on my body that I thought might have been a sign of skin cancer. Thank God it wasn't, but if it had been cancerous, it could have been a matter of life or death.

Through anointing, I'm in touch with my body and I've really gotten to know me. It's an empowering form of quality time that I look forward to. Needless to say, it was a conscious shift that I'm glad I made time for, as it continues to reward me—and ultimately those I care about—more than I can ever say.

Get Your Z's

I think sleep is the most awesome beauty treatment in the world—and believe me, I've tried enough treatments to know! I've found sleep to be the one balm that restores body, mind, and spirit and leaves them totally renewed at the end of the process. I've learned that the concept of "beauty sleep" is quite true, and when I skimp on it, I'm really cheating myself of one of the most transforming gifts God has given us. Sleep was determined by God to bring the day to a close, to refresh and recharge us, and most of all to empower us to be our best selves. Psalm 23 says "He maketh me to lie down"; well, just as sure as we get that wake-up call every morning, our bodies also alert us when it's time to rest. This intuition comes from our Creator, who knows our every need, which is why I've come to refer to it as that divine inspired period of healing. What I also know firsthand is that when we fail to heed this intuition, we compromise more than we know.

Experts say the majority of us need a full eight hours of sleep a night. And yet, according to the National Sleep Foundation, many are cheating themselves with less than six, skimming off this much-needed time-out that the body requires to heal from the stresses of everyday living. It seems we've become so adept at doing more on less, which is truly counterproductive, that we've forgotten what it feels like to be fully rested. As a result, many of us are carrying around what's known as a "sleep debt," trying to make it up on the weekends—or when our bodies are threatened with illness. We ignore the warning signs, such as a persistent cold we can't seem to kick, and continue to push ourselves to the max, because we don't see the connection between getting the proper rest and wellness. We also miss what I call those "blinking lights" that let us know that our sleep deprivation is affecting us in other ways: grouchiness, lack of concentration, reduced energy, headaches, poor posture, puffy or lackluster skin, dark circles, nail breakage, and hair loss. Not so obvious is what's going on behind the scenes: a weakened immune system and, over time, poor muscle tone. According to a 1996 research study published in the Journal of the Federation of American Societies of Experimental Biology, subjects who had their sleep cut in half had a significant reduction in the natural killer cells that combat infections and major diseases. Clearly the irony of sleep is that this passive state is highly productive! Those of us who are working at staying in shape also need to go to bed sooner rather than later. The muscle tone that we're striving for doesn't only depend on pressing weights at the gym: Human growth hormone (HGH), which promotes the growth, maintenance, and repair of healthy muscles, is released only during the deepest stages of sleep. It is said that the body passes through four stages nightly, with stage 1, which is referred to as the REM (rapid eye movement) period, being the lightest and stage 4 the deepest. It is during stages 3 and 4 that HGH is in the flow. So when we don't sleep enough hours, or when we wake up frequently during the night, we lose this much-needed deep sleep and deprive our bodies of sufficient quantities of this powerful hormone. We also deprive ourselves of the repair process that sleep effects on our skin and our immune system. Sleep cancels out the adverse effects of cortisol, a hormone that the body produces to maintain us during periods of stress; cortisol becomes a problem when increased levels of it are present in our bodies over long periods of time, as it compromises our immune system and, among other things, causes thinning of the skin.

Personally, I don't believe that a good night's rest is something that you turn off and on. I think of it as a restoring journey—one that I prepare to take every night so that I might receive all that it has to offer. To retreat into this sacred zone that allows me to rest and renew, I begin to put myself in the right frame of mind well before bedtime. I begin the moment I leave my office by emptying my mind of any thoughts associated with work and filling it with information that is calming, renewing, and affirming. When I arrive home, any work that I've brought along is deposited outside the bedroom for review the next morning. Then I give myself wholly to my family and the affairs of home until it's time for me to pay some serious attention to getting ready for bed—my time to attend solely to me and get ready to truly step away from the world in my sanctuary.

Because we spend nearly one-third of our lives sleeping, the environment to which we retreat should be an intimate, welcoming refuge that feeds the spirit. For singer Nancy Wilson, who says her bedroom is her favorite place for solitude, that means being surrounded by books that are dear to her. For talk-show host Star Jones, that means the most beautiful art and antiques. For me, coziness is paramount, and so everything in my room speaks to this aspect—from the choice of wallpaper (a soothing blue damask) to the subdued lighting, layers of select linens in subtle patterns, and sumptuous window treatments. Other essentials that say welcome include an antique settee at the foot of the bed and a vanity (my beautifying altar) for makeup, meditation, and Bible study. To me my bed-room is the most cherished space in our home, and the one I think of as a sanctuary because it's the place where I lay my burdens down, gain repose, and commune with God. Therefore, I put a lot of thought into making it the kind of room where I feel embraced in every way.

Experts have long said that our choices in color, furniture, decorations, and lighting can greatly influence our sleep patterns. Over the years, I've become quite sensitive to this and have developed a few practices that cause my bedroom to be the relaxing haven I desire. I refuse to use harsh overhead lighting unless I'm looking for an object, cleaning, or really need bright illumination for a specific task. Instead I utilize small, strategically placed table lamps to create the kind of glow I love. My senses are further seduced by scented candles, vases of dried flowers, pretty fragrance bottles, and transporting images. I also keep a selection of soothing jazz and environmental CDs within reach for the perfect sounds to drift off by. I complement these practices by dressing for "sleep success" in the dreamiest white cotton gowns with an antique feel or easy pajamas that drape coolly against my skin and make me feel totally pampered.

As tempting as all of these components are, nothing is more central to the journey than the vessel that transports us there: the bed. Made up with inviting linens, lots of comfy pillows, and perhaps a sachet of dried lavender awaiting you deep in your pillow, your bed extends an irresistible invitation to slumber in a welcoming cocoon. Think of your bed as a vessel that takes you on a restorative journey, and be sure that its foundation (mattress) is everything you need to set sail.

If stepping away from the world at large is a concern, think of investing in a canopy bed that will cradle you to sleep or a bed with an overhead frame like my daughter Samantha has, which allows her to close out the world with deeply colored drapes and therefore intimately drift off to sleep.

SLEEP TIGHT

To help you call it a night, here are some beauty-rest dos and don'ts:

DO

- Establish a sleep-inducing ritual, such as taking a warm bath or shower or tucking into bed with a great book of poetry

- Keep your bedroom well ventilated and around 68° Fahrenheit

- Invest in great sheets—delicious tones, patterns that seduce, and textures that invite—and keep in mind that the higher the thread count, the softer the sheet, so look for thread counts of 180–330

- If you have difficulty getting to sleep, try diverting your mind with some high-tech help by investing in a white-noise machine; to prevent complacency, get one that has a multiplicity of sounds, especially those associated with nature

DON'T

- Drink caffeinated beverages or alcohol before bed—though caffeine is a stimulant and alcohol is a depressant, both will fracture your sleep time

- Eat a heavy meal prior to retiring; digesting it will surely keep you from resting easy

- Work out late in the evening—allow five to six hours before bedtime, as exercise energizes as well as raises your body temperature, which causes alertness

- Watch television or work in bed

- Go to bed with a "full platter"—in other words, a busy mind

- Shortchange yourself when investing in a mattress

Today it seems like getting a full night's rest is a luxury, given the many demands on our personal time. However, wisdom dictates that we never view it as such. We must recognize sleep as the priority that it is: an important time for self that we must never skimp on.

Recharge Through Yoga

When I first met Bessie and Sadie Delany, they were 102 and 104 years old, respectively. They were sharp, witty, fiercely independent and doing yoga Monday through Friday! In fact, Sadie had been practicing yoga for about forty years; she had begun doing it with her mother in an effort to help straighten out her mother's posture. Later, when Bessie turned 80, she decided that Sadie looked better than her and joined her. I was floored; these elder sisters could do things with their bodies that I could only dream about! What also left an indelible impression on me was just how in tune they were with themselves. They had just completed their first book, *Having Our Say*, which was coauthored with Amy Hill Hearth, and it not only was filled with priceless observations of a lifetime but offered a real window on their wisdom, which to this day is humbling to me. The Delany sisters were centered, totally at peace with themselves, and fulfilled beyond a shadow of a doubt. It's no wonder their story went on to become a hit show on Broadway. What tenacity they had! And though they since have passed on from "labor to reward," as the elders say, they still serve as premier examples to me of two women who chose an empowering path in life and never deviated from it.

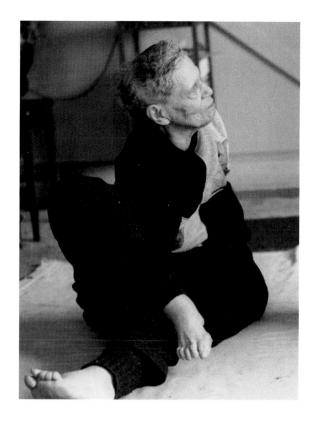

*Centenarian
Sadie Delany*

I'm sorry that I didn't ask them why they continued to practice yoga. I'm sure if I had, I would have gained some incredible insights about this discipline, which dates back over five thousand years. Then again, discipline might have been their reason for doing so. Yoga requires self-discipline, focus, and coordination—strengths they would never want to be without. It also requires that you remain fully in the moment as you move from one posture to another. What it gives in return is a gift beyond measure: harmony of mind, body, and spirit.

It is said that yoga retrains the mind and body to relax completely, which in turn allows the body to recharge. Other attributes include mental balance, improved concentration, stress reduction, relief from various physical tensions, and muscle and bone strengthening. What's also interesting is this observation from Frank Jude Boccio, D.Ay., yoga instructor at the Energy Center in Brooklyn, New York: "People [practicing] yoga begin to maintain a non-judgmental [attitude] and state of awareness [that allows them] to become less reactive. They develop more confidence and inner strength, as opposed to just body strength." Perhaps therein lies another reason why the Delany sisters continued to practice yoga. After all, they were two strong solo acts who moved and grooved through life at their own pace, making choice decisions about what mattered to their world and what didn't. Surprisingly enough, that excluded something many of us could not do without—telephones! They also never married, to which Bessie attributed the fact that they both lived past one hundred. What is most certain, though, is this truth: It had to have taken great confidence and strength to take the path they chose. I'm sure everything, including their devotion to practicing yoga, fortified them for the journey.

To me, yoga is a centering tool, one that I utilize whenever I feel I need to quietly reconnect. It's sort of like pushing the pause button on the world when it's too noisy, and realigning myself so I can deal. Staying in the present is a real challenge for me, but whenever I'm moving through yoga postures and taking those deep cleansing breaths, I'm totally caught up in the moment. Once I've completed the session, I feel so euphoric that it's almost like I've been to a spa! No surprises there—"different yoga postures release and cleanse," says Saeeda Hafiz, a certified yoga instructor in Pittsburgh, Pennsylvania. Hafiz likens yoga to an internal bath and adds, "Once you begin to cleanse the organs, use the breath to feed the cells, your mind begins to clear, you start to have more positive thoughts. You begin to connect to your body and who you are."

Ideally, you should look for yoga schools or centers that offer classes for beginners. You might also try out your first experience at a day or destination spa and then place yourself in a few workshop sessions at a center. What's important is to take a class that isn't too crowded so the instructor can give you the individual attention you may need. You should feel welcome, not intimidated, and you should leave each session inspired to return. This is about you getting more acquainted with you, so it's important that you feel fully supported. Here are some other points to keep in mind:

- Always wear comfortable clothes so you can move easily and so the instructor can monitor your body movements.

- Look for a cheery, softly lit, well-maintained space. Wooden floors are a must, as are top-quality mats, blankets, and possibly pillows for additional support.

- Make sure the location of the center you've chosen is convenient. You may end up attending class two or three times a week, so it should be easily accessible to your home or workplace. If frequency in attending classes is an issue for you, ask your instructor to recommend a suitable video that you can utilize in the privacy of your home.

- A classical yoga center should offer a blend of Iyengar (pose-oriented) and Ashtanga (movement-oriented) classes. Although there are many styles of yoga, the differences are usually about emphasis, such as focusing on strict alignment of the body, coordination of breath and movement, holding the postures, or flow from one posture to another. No one style is better than another—it's simply a matter of personal preference.

Boccio offers this encouragement: "Expose yourself to different interpretations with different teachers for a different point of view," and urges that we use yoga "as an opportunity to learn more about yourself."

Reconnect Through Tai Chi

Mind-body fitness expert Fran Sachs, of the Sea Change Healing Center in New York City, introduced me briefly to a few martial arts exercises while we were working out one day, and from that point on I became quite curious. I was impressed by the sense of well-being and control I felt after practicing what was simply a series of focused movements, and so I wanted to discover more. One day during a visit to Lake Austin Spa and Resort in Austin, Texas, I took advantage of this desire by taking a class in tai chi, an ancient Chinese martial art. Designed to increase balance, strength, flexibility, and circulation, tai chi is a centuries-old strain of meditation and movement that gives the mind a chance to connect to the body. It causes you to slow down and get in tune with yourself through a rhythmic series of flowing, circular movements and focused breath work. Like yoga, it also teaches you how to pull out of the fast-forward pace of everyday living and just be present in the moment. Taking this class made me realize I hadn't been challenged like this since I was a child! Little did I know how uncoordinated I had become, or how much I needed to strengthen that virtue known as patience. Tai chi helps you to master both.

One of the things I love the most about tai chi, aside from the fact that it's another way to spend time with myself, is its emphasis on correct posture—something I continually have to work at. Chinese healers believe that bad posture impedes the flow of chi (energy) and causes tension as well as back problems and shallow breathing. There was a time in my life when I could relate to all of these implications, and so I now personally believe this to be true. Practicing tai chi causes you to align your body correctly by keeping your knees slightly bent, therefore releasing tension from them and other parts of your body. It's an expertise that doesn't happen overnight, but through regular practice and an abiding consciousness, you can come to assume this correct form.

I had experienced trouble with my lower back for a long time. There were even times when I was dependent on a chiropractor. Sometimes life gives us signs and we just ignore them—we keep having the same mental conversations with ourselves and diminishing those signals in the process. But I agree with Sheryl Lee Ralph, who told me one day to realize when you need a change and allow these signs to cause you to consider yourself. Slowly but surely, I realized that I didn't want to have a relationship with a chiropractor! I desired to be in control of my vessel and to do those things that would nurture it and keep it in top form. I had been coached a long time ago about correct form, but I didn't keep those instructions at the top of my mind. Today I am more conscious and have since taken lessons from a trainer to not only improve my posture but strengthen my abdominal muscles, which play a great role in supporting the back. Now I no longer experience distress in this area. My thinking has changed too. When I think about form now, the term *carriage* comes to mind, and with that a beautiful visual of our sisters in the Motherland who proudly stride through the marketplace balancing baskets on their heads. This ability denotes more than physical strength; it communicates a strong sense of self, character, and internal balance—the very tools we need to stride through life purposefully while balancing whatever challenges it brings our way!

Satisfy Your Kneads

Massage is one of the greatest forms of natural healing of all time. Whether you're seeking to de-stress, ease muscle tension, soothe arthritis, or be rejuvenated, there's a specific massage technique designed to deliver. To me, given both the hectic pace of daily life and the fact that we've become such a low-touch society, massage has become more essential to our well-being than ever before. Personally, I can't say enough about its restorative benefits. Depending on my needs—to unwind, to ease the very real symptoms of PMS, or to erase the painful stress that settles across my shoulders from long periods at the computer—there's a form of massage with my name on it! In particular, I love having what's known as a lymphatic drainage massage, which I use specifically to reduce water retention prior to my menstrual period. According to Brenda L. Griffith, president-elect of the American Massage Therapy Association, located in Evanston, Illinois, this form of massage in the hands of a qualified therapist is also excellent for the edema often experienced by breast cancer survivors: "It's incredibly beneficial to them in draining the additional fluids that come after surgery." I'm also deeply conscious of the many other physical and psychological benefits of this formalized power of touch. I remember a time when my mother was hospitalized and recovering from a mild heart attack. During that period I would massage her feet and legs as well as her hands each day, and I'm convinced that it played a significant role in her recovery, although I couldn't put my finger on *why* until I spoke with Griffith. "When you go through an illness like that you're being poked, prodded, and touched, but not in a positive way. It's an uncertain time; these are

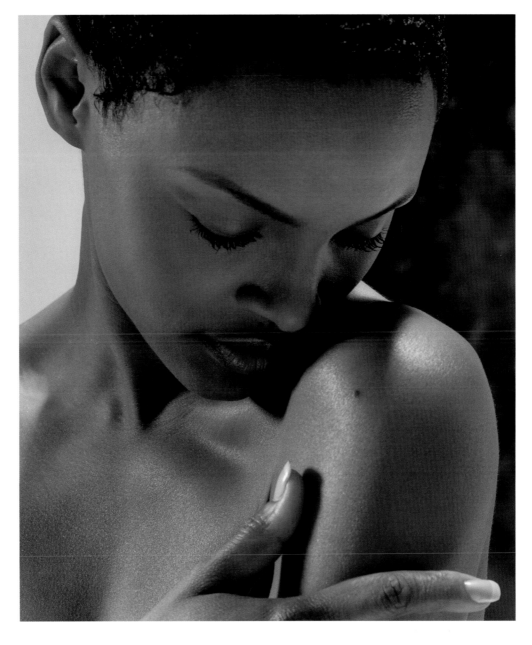

not people you know that are touching you, and so massage brings back the idea of a loving, nurturing touch, one that's not in the regimen that you're experiencing at that time, and the mental side of that is invaluable in the recovery process," she told me. While I'm not suggesting that anyone substitute massage for medical care—in fact, according to Christel Alkana, a polarity wellness educator and certified massage therapist at the Body Clinic in Los Angeles, if you're on certain medications such as blood thinners, have high blood pressure, or are undergoing chemotherapy, massage is definitely inadvisable—I clearly understand that it can play a role in increased well-being. Another time to forgo a massage is when you're coming down with a cold or the flu. Having a massage during this stage of the illness is detrimental because, as Alkana explains, "you're

*Model
Lisa Butler*

increasing the circulation and spreading the virus." So it's best to wait until you know you're on the road to recovery. It's always wise to check with your doctor if you have a medical condition or even suspect a concern. For example, if you're diabetic, he or she may okay a massage, but only a very light one, such as a Swedish massage. So consulting your practitioner in these and other instances is the only way to have a massage free of concern.

What's key about massage, beyond its obvious feel-good factor, is its impact on your emotional beauty. First of all, it reduces what the experts call the "fight-or-flight response," brought on by stress. If you've ever caught yourself in the mirror with your shoulders hunched as if you're suspended on a line, you know what I mean! Internally, what this means is that stress hormones are surging, your muscles are tight, and, over time, your heart is being taxed and your immune system weakened. Massage reverses the process. According to Griffith, more and more studies are proving what stress does to our bodies. She points out, "Given the fact that massage helps with stress reduction and relaxation, you have a way to fight illness, be stronger, and help the immune system function the way it was meant to function." How does it work? "By enhancing the blood flow, we're also enhancing the flow of the lymph system, which carries the antibodies that help us fight off disease," says Griffith, who's also a massage veteran with a private practice in Richmond, Virginia. On top of that, it boosts the output of endorphins, mood-elevating and pain-dulling brain chemicals, which is why you feel so good and so relaxed when you get off the massage table. These are reasons why, depending on the season in your life, a massage may be as essential as a mammogram—only *you* know the score. This is why I suggest that we not consider a massage a practice for only the rich and famous, nor a gift that you're deserving of simply on your birthday or Mother's Day. Your wellness and inner harmony may dictate having one weekly or monthly. And these considerations might also call for you to mix it up when it comes to the type of massage you get, whether it be a Swedish massage (to relax your muscles and increase blood flow) or a sports massage (which, by the way, isn't just for athletes)! "A sports massage is perfect for those weekend warriors, the people who go out and rake leaves for eight hours and can't figure out why their neck and shoulders hurt. They can benefit greatly, as can someone who goes out for a power walk for the first time and doesn't warm up, as they can have the same injuries and the same response to that as an athlete could," adds Griffith.

And the benefits of massage are far more practical in our everyday lives than we know. The passionate Griffith points out its very beneficial effects for widows, divorcees, and singles who don't have relatives close by. "Who's touching them?" she asks. "They might get a handshake or a touch at church on Sunday, but there's nobody touching their bodies in a loving, respectful, nurturing way that says *I care*," which is essential.

It's important to also realize that you play a role in how beneficial your massage will be. According to Blanche Williams Cory, who's nationally certified in therapeutic massage and bodywork, "effectiveness and communication between the massage therapist and the client go hand in hand," so it's important to be specific about your needs and desires when stepping away for this curative experience. "Let the therapist know you've had a rough day, and that'll get you a soothing massage. If you work out every day and are dealing with muscle soreness, or if you don't have good mobility in certain areas, that'll tell the therapist something else," she says. Most of all, Williams Cory, whose audio book *You and Your Power: Making the Connection* is used at national health institutes and retreats to help both therapists and those who are looking to manage their well-being understand massage more deeply, says the most important consideration to keep in mind is that massage therapists are there to create an environment that is conducive for the clients to heal themselves. So I urge you to see massage as another way to listen within and then make the appropriate response with the healing power of touch.

If you find that you can't visit a massage therapist each and every time the need arises, learn how to give yourself a massage. There are many tools available to assist you, from foot massagers to those specifically designed for the shoulders and back. You can also borrow from some of the simpler techniques used by the pros. One of my favorites involves massaging my temples with small circles using a minty massage lotion. I find this helps to relieve tension and ease the occasional

DIFFERENT STROKES

If you're looking to explore the different types of massage and body work, here's a briefing on those most widely available and their benefits:

SWEDISH A very light, soothing massage, using very long strokes; aids in overall relaxation, stimulates circulation, relieves knotty muscles (depending on the pressure used).

DEEP TISSUE Uses a very firm, focused pressure, often concentrating on specific areas of the body; for muscle soreness, as it releases toxins and lactic acid (which builds up in the muscles) and increases circulation.

SHIATSU A type of bodywork that works on the body's pressure points to improve energy flow; alleviates chronic fatigue, anxiety, and pain, relieves stress.

SPORTS MASSAGE A rigorous massage similar to deep tissue massage; utilized for specific muscular aches; removes toxins, relieves soreness.

REFLEXOLOGY Involves using the fingers to apply pressure to reflex points specifically on the hands and feet; assists the body in bringing its systems into balance, improves circulation, aids in depression, counters stress.

AROMATHERAPY Incorporates the use of essential oils with a base oil to enhance the massage; releases tension.

HOT STONE Uses smooth heated stones, combined with oil and gliding strokes; relaxes, soothes muscle soreness.

To find a licensed massage therapist in your area, contact the American Massage Therapy Association at 888-843-2682 or www.amtamassage.org, or ask your health care professional for a recommendation.

migraine before it becomes overwhelming. To help you get started, try a few of the self-massage moves listed below, from Williams Cory. And as you go through the techniques, remember to be mindful of breathing deeply from your diaphragm. "Part of our job is to have the right intention," she says, and asks us to say to ourselves during this time for self: *I'm breathing in relaxation and I'm breathing out stress; I'm breathing in peace and I'm breathing out conflict!*

SHOULDERS Take your right hand, cup it around the fleshy portion of your left shoulder (the area that bridges your neck and outer shoulder), where tension stakes a claim. Squeeze and hold for at least seven seconds, counting in your mind while breathing deeply in and out, and then release. Repeat the movement four or five times, and then administer the same process to the other shoulder.

For an added benefit, you can follow this one up by soaking a hand towel in comfortably hot water, wringing it out, and applying it across the area—or heat an organic spa pillow or wrap in the microwave and do the same.

FEET Sit on the floor or on your bed, Indian style, and take one foot into your hands, making sure the sole of your foot is pointing upward. Place both of your thumbs on the foot just under the big toe and apply pressure. Continue the motion across the toe line and then repeat up the middle of the foot and finally along the arch.

LEGS Sit cross-legged on the floor or on your bed. Using a massage oil, begin by alternating squeezing and kneading your calves. Work your way up to the thighs, first on one leg and then onto the other.

Hit the Spa!

Another way to halt time and tend to self is to visit a spa. Whether you've got an hour, a day, or time for a pack-the-bags retreat, this beautifying escape is one I urge you to make room for. To me, stepping away to rejuvenate body, mind, and spirit is an example of wisdom at work in our lives. More than any treat for a special occasion, visiting a spa represents temple management, and no one is more deserving of this supreme care than you! What I've learned from experience is that just when you think you don't have time for it is when you need it the most. I'm not ashamed to tell you that I have visited a day spa in the midst of a truly hectic day at work and come back all the more centered and ready for any challenge just because of that time to be nurtured and gain focus. I didn't always feel this way, however; in fact it took me a while to get over the guilt of indulging myself in the midst of pressure or of taking time away from the family for such a seemingly personal benefit. But I learned the error of such thinking and began to put things in perspective and value my need to be *stroked.* Now I know it's essential to balancing a busy life, giving of oneself, and maintaining well-being. Oprah Winfrey says, "My good sister friend who's also the executive producer of my show suggested a couple of years ago that we build a spa at the studio and I said that is the most ridiculous idea I ever heard—what are we going to do with a spa? And she said we're going to go to the spa and take care of ourselves. We now have a Harpo Spa (full service) which has been one of the greatest, luxurious, and seductive gifts that we have given to ourselves. We have a production company that is predominantly women and we work very hard and we found it difficult for women to take care of themselves. So now we have a respite, an oasis to go to in the middle of the day. And I was probably the last person in the building to take advantage of it,

■ **Spa Finders is an agency that specializes in helping you find the perfect destination or day spa. Log on to www.spafinders.com, or call 1-800-ALL-SPAS; if you're looking for a day spa, be sure to use the Web site locator.**

■ **The International Spa Association (ISPA) offers a spa locator service at www.experienceispa.com; from there, proceed to "Search for a Spa."**

■ **For information on the Odyssey Network or reservations, check out idamar.com or call 1-800-277-1311.**

because I felt guilty, in the middle of the day having a massage. But what I found is giving back to myself allows me to have more to give to the rest of the world. I speak to women around the world and my message is that we are all responsible for our lives. So you have to take care of yourself so that you will be in a better position to take care of others." I've personally become a sponge for learning what's going to better yours truly, whether it's an oxygen facial or a different perspective when it comes to nutritional counseling. So I not only have those routine visits at my favorite day spas, but include time at those sanctuaries otherwise known as "destination spas," where I can really turn off the stress and be restored. I especially love getting away to those retreats where the emphasis is on treating the *whole* person, like my junket to Odyssey Network, an annual spa conference for women of color that includes visits to various types of desert spas, along with adventurous activities and empowerment sessions over the course of several days. The payoff here is learning good habits to incorporate into my lifestyle, from stress management to healthy eating, so I can deal on both the personal and professional levels. Other times I enjoy heading off to those spas that specialize in the gift of solitude—along with the pampering treats one might expect, there's a big focus on spiritual restoration, maintaining well-being, and, again, time for self. Many times these are the spas where phones *aren't* available in your room, where the treatments are more organic, and the sessions, which often take place in natural surroundings, are centered on soul-searching techniques. These experiences are on their way to becoming prescriptive in my life.

After filming *Introducing Dorothy Dandridge*, actress Halle Berry told me she went on a big spa adventure herself to buff, puff, and start anew. She says, "Spiritually, I had time alone with myself even though someone else was present. I had time to reflect on where I've been and let Dorothy go, because she had become so much a part of my being during the work, so it was time to let her go and for Halle to come back." Berry also told me she saw this time as a way for her to begin to face whatever her next challenge would be. Little did she know there was an Oscar-winning role in her future, one that would cause her to prove herself to those who doubted her capabilities.

The old saying "A change of scene will do you good" is still true. So make sure to pencil yourself in and hit the spa as part of your plan to spend time with yourself. And please don't wait for a special occasion, because when you get right down to it, you're more than worthy of being nurtured *every day*. I know that, like me, you don't skip a beat when it comes to caring for others, so all I'm saying is be sure to include yourself in the plan.

My Ten-Point Anti-Stress Plan for Life

We are all familiar with the old adage "If you fail to plan, you plan to fail." Given modern life's increasing responsibilities upon us as women, as well as the opportunities we'll want to seize, it is clear to me that the only way for us to lead a balanced life is with a plan—one that considers time for self as par for the course. Without a doubt, stress, no matter what shape or form, not only alters the quality of our lives, but is a culprit at the heart of many an illness requiring continuous medical care. What I've learned from personal experience, as well as the many sisters I've talked to, is that tending to self is an essential form of preservation that maintains your entire being and enables you to keep everything in perspective. This healthy, emotionally in-touch approach to life can serve to prevent stress from causing serious concern in our lives. Moreover, when your life is in balance, I find that you are fully able to handle stress, as opposed to allowing it to handle you.

The ten points listed below bolster my body, mind, and spirit and keep them in perfect harmony. They also serve as a checklist to help me get back on track during those times when I may feel off-balance or especially stressed. Through careful review, I can see if I've neglected any of these points or haven't given them the recognition they deserve. I look at it this way: God's intention is for us to live an abundant life, and if we're experiencing anything less, we're living beneath our privilege!

TAKE TEN:

1   *Recognize that God is in control.* Scripture says, "He that keepeth thee shall neither slumber nor sleep." So don't try to take over—God has not only your back but every aspect of you! The goal, then, is to be convinced and fully assured that God wants only the best for you. Our elders put it this way: "Let go and let God." That's the first point of defense against stress on the path to total well-being.

2   *Know your value.* And give evidence by committing to what honors you, such as centering rituals that will restore you, as opposed to practices that only deplete you and keep you from being your best. After every major accomplishment, be sure to give yourself an *emotional* break before moving on to the next big thing, and use this time to reflect and recharge. Stay focused; remember that those with a high self-esteem gain their approval from within and not from outside sources. Last but not least, seek to please your Creator, who made you in His image and whose instruction is there to affirm you throughout life and in every experience. This will keep you from wandering off track and losing sight of what's really important.

3   *Be grandiose in your appraisal of your total well-being.* God intended for us to experience an abundant life—that means an existence far greater than we could ever expect, rich in value and rejuvenating of our entire being. Our role therefore is to regard ourselves with a Godly love, and that means that we cherish and take care of ourselves to the best of our ability, inside and out. It also means working in what experts call a "cooperative spirit," where you don't add to the stress of daily living by overtaxing yourself, but rather assign reasonable priority to those goals you'd like to accomplish. Anything beyond this thinking is really a compromise of all that we have to offer.

4   *Affirm yourself.* Exercise body, mind, and spirit to the highest level daily. The Bible says, "Faith without works is dead." This means there's work for us to do! And know that affirming your entire self has its rewards. Not only will it allow you to move in this world with stress under your control, it will empower you to stay on track and, most of all, give you discernment about what is really worth having. It will also motivate you to choose quality time with yourself above the quantity of things you can possess. Finally, make certain to surround yourself with positive people whose love and encouragement will fortify your efforts.

5   *Keep gratitude in the flow.* Whatever the season is in your life, and regardless of whether the stress that accompanies it is great or small, recognize that you have so much to be thankful for. You see, our purpose in life is altered only by the things that we allow to have control over us. The Creator instructs us "to be temperate in all things." So we have to ask ourselves, "Will this last forever?" Chances are the answer is a resounding no! So take the perspective of your elders by being confident

58

SELF-SEDUCTION

that this too shall pass. And in the process, let's be sure to count our blessings instead of allowing stress to rule our outlook. That's a sure way to remain in control.

6   *Commune with yourself.* Keep your mind's eye open and fine-tuned by spending time with yourself in ways that allow you to relax, look within, and fully examine where you are. Meditate, practice yoga (another great way to hear yourself), express your heart in a journal, and by all means stay on the path of self-discovery, which in and of itself is higher ground. This will help you to harness stress in all of its forms—from the tension that can accompany a rigorous schedule to simply that of an anxious mind. Equally important, keep your inner dialogue with yourself positive; speak those things to yourself that will encourage you to be powerful, so that you can graciously meet every challenge.

7   *Pamper thyself.* This is an enriching imperative. Making sure to take the time to nurture ourselves will keep us from being on the edge and allow us to see the light at the end of the tunnel in all circumstances. Routine nurturing of body, mind, and spirit will also allow you to rise above stress, as opposed to allowing it to engulf you and cause you to lose your perspective. Make pampering yourself more than a notion—make it a way of life. You are more than worthy!

8   *Don't skimp on sleep.* Sleep is meant to bring the day to a close and to give our body, mind, and spirit a much-needed respite. When we cheat on sleep, we're only cheating ourselves by cutting short this divine-inspired period of healing. We also cut short our ability to withstand stress by remaining calm and focused, as our inner reserves are compromised from lack of rest. So make getting the proper amount of sleep part of your plan to de-stress.

9   *Celebrate yourself!* Do something each and every day that brings you joy. Scripture tells us that joy is an important fruit of the spirit; if you think about it, it is joy that refreshes us and causes us to see the glass as half full as opposed to half empty. What I've also found is that joy and stress cannot coexist, so I make certain to integrate practices that give me joy on a daily basis—it's my way of "hanging in there," as the expression goes. So I allow myself to have fun and to enjoy pursuits that bring pleasure into my life. Most of all, I've come to learn that a large part of celebrating yourself has a lot to do with how well you treat others, and so joy has

become more meaningful to me through those acts of kindness that I extend to those I come in contact with.

10 *Enlist the power of prayer.* Remember, the secret to checking stress is to treat yourself as an integral whole, in the highest order. To do this, you need a power source, a generator, to give you the constant support you'll need as well as a channel of connection. I think of prayer as the channel and God as my generator. Prayer is what allows me to stay the course, to rise above the fray and keep running when I'd rather sit down. The wisdom of the scriptures dictates that we remain in constant contact with our Creator in order to realize our best selves. When we fail to do so, we short-circuit and give stress free rein in our lives. So make sure to keep the lines of prayer in the flow so that you can put stress in its proper place—beneath you!

Staying the Course

Just the thought of passing time at the ocean's edge, waves lapping at my toes and listening to what's on my heart, is a restorative desire I want to realize more and more. But we all know real life isn't like that! So the keeper is to order your steps so that the peace and understanding that come by way of moments like that are a regular part of the journey. Like Halle, I believe that nurturing time is one of the first steps to loving yourself. "When you're able to spend time alone with yourself, then you are truly empowered," says the busier-than-busy actress, who also pointed out that without this capability you're "beholden to other people for your happiness, and that's giving away too much control!" So learn to cherish the time you have to give yourself, and if you still have trouble making it a reality, take the advice of Dr. Magdoff, who urges us to treat ourselves the way we treat other people. She suggests we begin by giving thought to these questions: How would we treat a friend? Would we really spend so little time with her? "There's always a good reason to not be spending the time, and unfortunately guilt is a big motivator," she adds. But let's agree that allowing this to keep us from this intimate approach to self-care will no longer be an option.

Now, you and I know all too well that change is one thing, and commitment to it is something else entirely! After September 11, we all made promises not to take life for granted. Let's not slip back into the old ways but continue to rise and walk in the newness of a life that we won't fail to appreciate ever again. For sure, as you formulate your plan of action to nurture yourself, challenges will come and, if you're not careful, force you off track. Maintaining a sense of commitment and a realistic approach will keep you from going there. So plot your course and get on with it! To help, here are some ideas to keep time for self in your life a way of being that's here to stay:

- Affirm that time to nurture your physical and emotional beauty is a necessity that you won't neglect because it not only benefits you personally but also benefits your family, friends, and all those you touch.

- Keep your goals realistic and start small. Think about those things that you would love to do or wish were true in your life, whether it's a weekly paraffin manicure or time to take lunch in the park. Then get out your calendar and schedule it just as you would any other appointment, medical, social, or otherwise—and keep it!

- View even your daily rituals as a way to spend time with yourself and find small ways to enhance the experience. For example, don't just wash your hair—turn it into something more by using an aromatherapy cleanser, formulated to balance, cleanse, and restore you from head to toe!

- Stay focused on the life you are trying to live, so it doesn't elude you.

- Share your goals with your family and friends so they can encourage you in this necessary endeavor. You'll need their support, as privately held goals are easy to lose sight of.

- Don't take on too many goals at once. Pace yourself, so these changes can become a way of life for you, as opposed to a short-term promise.

- Keep a record of your progress in your journal, all the while adding new suggestions and describing how and when you plan to achieve them.

- As you move forward, keep deepening your commitment, and if you do fall off track, don't pause there—get right back in the flow!

- Be willing to go the distance to reach your goals, whether it means rising earlier or, if you're a mom, exchanging child-sitting opportunities with a friend or scheduling an activity for the children.

- Try something new—whether it's a hot-air balloon ride or a hot stone massage. As you move forward, make an effort to explore those practices that will both deepen your beauty and move you further along on the path to self-discovery.

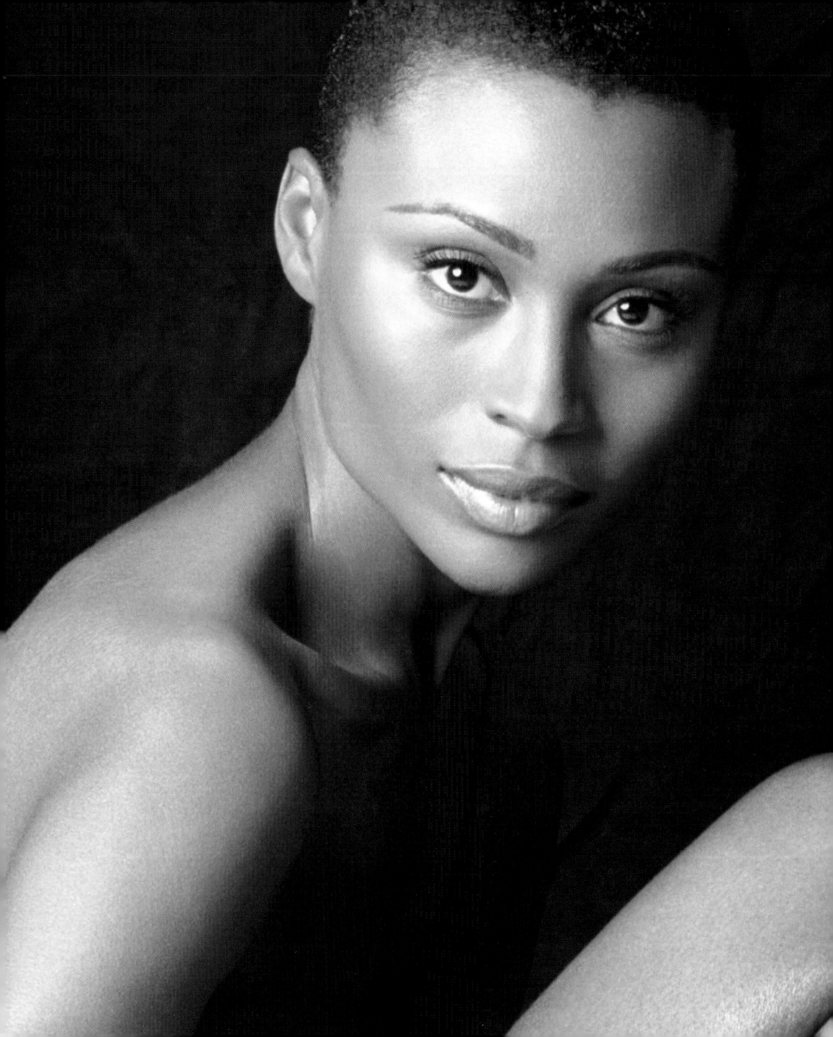

3 THE SKIN YOU'RE IN

"She knows who she is
because she knows
who she isn't."

NIKKI GIOVANNI, POET

As a child, I was in and out of the doctor's office for more skin allergies than he probably had listed in his manual! To this day, I get a real laugh when I think about the time when my family had wall-to-wall carpet laid, only to have it taken up the next day because I was allergic to it! I'm sure it wasn't funny to them. I think to keep her sense of composure, my mother was always on the lookout for advice that might help *both* of us. She told me once that she and the late Nat King Cole, whom my mother knew through Sarah Vaughan, used to trade stories about me and his daughter Natalie, as it seemed she too had skin concerns growing up. (Of course you wouldn't know that by looking at Cole's gorgeous skin today!) By the time I reached my tweens, my mother began to show me the paces of caring for my skin, which by then had started to settle down, although new food allergies had shown up to take its place. I was more than interested, as my mother tended her skin with the kind of prestige products that I couldn't wait to get my hands on—which I made certain to do every time she went out. So at thirteen I knew all the tricks and practices, from how to take your makeup off with cold cream to, unfortunately, what a bleaching cream could do!

By the time I reached high school, I thought of myself as an accomplished maven when it came to skin care, because of my ever-curious nature as well as the many lessons at my mother's side. My mother knew herself inside and out, and she never deviated from her truth. This was especially so when it came to taking care of her skin. By the time she made her transition in 1994, at 67, her skin was smooth, supple, and glowing in a way that I have yet to know. Of the lessons she taught me, the greatest was to know the skin you're in. She always put great emphasis on being clear about what belonged to you; in fact, this was her mantra for everything, from boyfriends to clothing. So even though it took me a while to apply this thinking across the board, I got it.

This advice is the same that I offer to you. And it's what I see at work in the lives of women who've taken charge of their skin to the best of their ability. We all know how frustrating it is when skin isn't what you desire it to be. It can be a real esteem breaker, especially in an image-conscious country such as the United States, where people make their determinations about you based on how you look long before you ever open your mouth. Unfair? Yes. But as makeup artist Jay Manuel says, "That's the real down-low."

What I find to be true is that more than we may think comes under the umbrella known as "care," and these modern times call for us to be well informed about what is in our control, and aware of all the things that can have a direct impact on our skin. Part of caring for my skin includes exercising three times a week and juicing fresh vegetables and fruits five days a week to boost my intake of antioxidants. Years ago I wouldn't have made either connection. But I'm clear that exercise puts a luminosity on my face that's *not* fleeting, and it tones and strengthens my body in the process. Experts say that exercise increases blood flow to the skin, and when it's combined with a healthy, balanced diet full of antioxidant-rich foods (antioxidants neutralize unstable molecules known as free radicals, which attack healthy cells) as well as healthy fats to keep skin hydrated and promote cell renewal, the surface of the skin will stay looking fresh. This is not a bit of news I would have associated with skin care practices early on, but now I do, and so I want you too to think "out of the jar." Since I've talked with nutritionist Oz Garcia, author of *The Healthy High Tech Body*, who helps women I admire—like model Veronica Webb—micromanage their beauty, I believe that there is a reason why our sisters whose diets consist of broiled fish, fresh vegetables, and fruits— like in some parts of the Motherland and in places like the Mediterranean and Asia—have beautiful, glowing skin. "You cannot disregard the fact that eating a typical American diet that is hormonally challenging you isn't going to positively affect the quality of your skin—it's going to contribute to acne and pimples, and make you lose color in your skin whether you're a Black woman or an Asian woman," says Garcia, who urges us to support ourselves with foods that nurture the skin from within. "Because everything is connected," as he says and as my mother taught me, you have to know what belongs to you and, more importantly, treat it accordingly.

About Face

When it comes to the skin's surface, most of us know that we need to treat and protect it. But some of the greatest care you can give your skin happens internally. Today, many experts suggest that clear, radiant skin has more to do with how you manage your life than what you apply to the skin's surface. Proper rest, diet, and exercise all play a role in its behavior and appearance. After all, our skin is the largest barometer of what is going on in our bodies, both physically and emotionally. It even reveals our secret faux pas, such as smoking, drinking, overindulging in caffeinated beverages, and soaking up the sun.

All this is not to say that there aren't factors beyond our control that play a role in its appearance. Genetics figure into the picture greatly, but how you build upon them does as well. Conditions such as acne, which can strike without any warning (even at 35), and other troublesome concerns such as hyperpigmentation, excessive oiliness, dryness, and even allergies can all mar the skin. And eczema and psoriasis can and do wreak havoc on our skin as well as our nerves. But I believe your best complexion is achieved by paying close attention to your inner health and your lifestyle and by adopting a sensible, informed care regimen that includes being attentive to your skin and what it's saying to you as well as consulting the appropriate experts. Ultimately, by managing your skin from the inside out, understanding its personality as well as making the right choices in terms of care, products, and professional support, you'll be able to achieve and maintain your best complexion for keeps.

Skin IQ

There is nothing, *nothing* more important when it comes to beauty basics than understanding *your* skin and its behavior patterns. There's a constantly running dialogue that lets you know whether your skin is calm and happy, stressed, or in trouble. I was amused when actress LaTanya Richardson Jackson told me her skin was going through what she deemed as a "needy personality" phase. "It not only lets me know it's there, it'll turn on me too if I've been remiss, and say, 'How about this, Miss Good Skin—a couple of pimples!'" The busy actress cites this as her skin's way of claiming her attention. My combination skin responds to the power of touch and loves to be massaged and nourished with essential extracts that balance and further tone up its radiance, like those in the cleansers I use for makeup removal. This action also stimulates the circulation and makes my nightly application of a vitamin C moisturizer really pay off, allowing me to wake up with a nice glow that lasts throughout the day.

*Actress
LaTanya Richardson
Jackson*

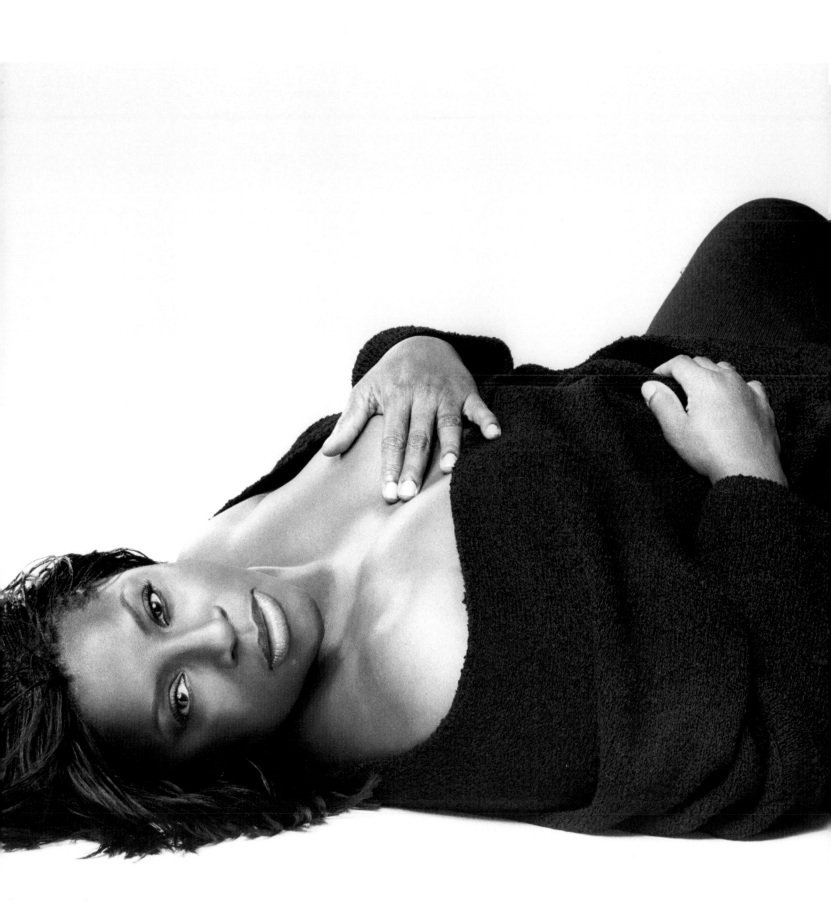

Our skin has lifestyle and care habits as well as product types that it favors, and learning to read its response is all part of claiming and maintaining our skin at its best. Understanding it begins with identifying your skin type. Start by washing your face and waiting thirty minutes, then check it against the following characteristics:

DRY Taut, has an ashy cast; white flakes, feels itchy, shows tiny surface lines

OILY Shiny, produces more sebum than average; feels slick, prone to breakouts and acne, large pores

COMBINATION Oily in the T-zone (forehead, nose, and chin), dry on the sides; breaks out occasionally

SENSITIVE Easily irritated, itchy; often dry and has a tendency to be blotchy

NORMAL Smooth and supple; balanced

Once you have determined your skin type, think of this information as your skin's basic ID. Now you're ready to establish a care regimen that will nurture your skin and keep it healthy. Be discerning when selecting products, and don't fall for lofty claims—remember, if something sounds too good to be true, it usually is. And don't be fooled into misreading your skin by buying into such myths as oily skin doesn't need a moisturizer. Says Iman, who rules over two skin care and cosmetic brands that address the needs and desires of women of color, "This isn't true—oily skin needs an *oil-free* moisturizer, it doesn't need an astringent." Shop for products for your skin type, not because they are new or make great claims, and make sure you avoid those with such skin-unfriendly ingredients as lanolin, mineral oil, fragrance, and alcohol. I also suggest that you start small—don't invest in a full line of skin care products and all its accessory items initially. Start with the most basic items, including cleanser, moisturizer, and eye balm or cream, and allow your skin to tell you if these are the products that fit comfortably. This way, if one or more of them don't, you'll be more easily able to determine which one is the offender and take it back for an exchange or refund. This is why it's important to spend your hard-earned dollars in places that will afford you this courtesy. If you find, however, that you really want to try something and returns aren't a part of the store's policy, then ask for samples, and don't be shy—request an amount that will allow you to experience the product for a few days, which will be enough time to see whether it works or if you have a reaction to it. Once you've settled on the basics, you can then look into those products that will go the extra mile to help you achieve added benefits or check small flare-ups as need be.

From there, it's important to watch your skin's behavior and learn to read its response to what you're sending it. If you suddenly break out one day, question the source and examine the look of the pimples instead of automatically reaching for products addressing acne—you may save your skin in the process by not being too hasty. If it persists, that's the time to see an expert you trust. Anything could have aggravated this concern, from a new hair product to a different laundry detergent—even fillers in a vitamin supplement (for more information see "Support Strategies for Special Concerns").

Your primary role here is to be diligent in caring for your skin by committing to a ritual that it loves. Here are some basic steps:

- *Come clean.* Washing your face with the appropriate cleanser to remove dead skin cells, pollution, and makeup, is a twice-daily bit of TLC it needs.

    OILY SKIN or acne-prone skin means you should look to an oil-free gel or soap formulated specifically for your skin type that has antibacterial ingredients as well as those that check oil without stripping your skin. You can consider those with alpha-hydroxy or salicylic acid if they're recommended by an expert. Oily skin hates to be scrubbed or stripped—it goes into defense mode when this happens, producing even more oil! Keep your actions gentle and your product choices cooperative.

    DRY SKIN dictates a mild, hydrating, creamy cleanser with milder surfactants and moisturizers that cleanse without drying out the skin. Dry skin likes to be "babied" with gentle strokes and warm—never hot—water when rinsed, and don't forget to pat, not rub, dry.

    COMBINATION SKIN calls for a gel, creamy cleansers that foam, or a bar specifically designed to thoroughly clean without stimulating oil production or clogging pores. Combination skin likes a happy medium, with cleansers that check and balance plus lots of clarifying water rinses.

    SENSITIVE SKIN needs products that have the least amount of preservatives and are fragrance-free (not unscented, which means they can contain a masking scent), dermatologist-tested, moisturizing, and extremely gentle. Depending on your degree of sensitivity, you may want a soapless cleanser or a mild glycerin bar. Sensitive skin dictates that you skip all exfoliators, fruit acids, enzymes, and products containing alcohol.

- *Nurture.* Many state-of-the-art cleansers now allow us to skip the toning phase and move on to the nurturing phase of a regimen—*moisturization.*

There are times when life seems to be on overload for all of us. Part of my coping strategy is to go back to the Word for a bit of encouragement and maybe an example or two of instruction for the stress that comes my way. Sometimes my best maneuver is to metaphorically imitate Jesus and move on, removing myself from what's at hand, as he did that day on the shores of the Sea of Galilee at Capernaum when he simply got in the boat and went over to the other side. I heard my minister say one day that when a challenge is too big for us, it's just right for God! So I'm learning to "give over," as the elders say, and I get this lesson more and more as I travel on this journey called life.

What baffles me to this day, however, is that there are those who continue to maintain that stress has no connection to any skin conditions other than eczema or psoriasis. To me there ought to be universal clarity on this subject! According to Dr. Susan Taylor, director of the Skin of Color Center at St. Luke's–Roosevelt Hospital in New York City, there is a very strong relationship between the skin (and hair) and stress. "Many of my patients who are under stress will report a flare-up of acne," adds Taylor. I remember clearly when the effects of stress would show up on my skin. I ended up going to a dermatologist, who told me it was directly related to stress, prescribed a cream, and basically told me that it would go away if I used the prescription as instructed. He didn't have to tell me that I needed to do my part and process the stress differently—that was self-evident. I later learned that one of my supervisors had the same condition, and right then and there, that told me that something was wrong with this picture. Well, I made up my mind that this wasn't going to be true of me, as I wasn't interested in suffering, nor was I being compensated financially to carry the load! To this day I am more than happy that the doctor didn't misdiagnose the problem, because I wasn't interested in having a relationship with a dermatologist over a great mystery!

According to Dr. Howard Murad, assistant professor of dermatology at the University of California at Los Angeles, your skin is just one portion of your body that's connected to every other portion of it, so if you have emotional stress, it's going to show up on your skin. For example, when you have a number of stressors going on, your body has to produce adrenaline to keep you going. "Adrenaline is produced in the adrenal glands, and in the adrenal glands is another hormone called DHEA, which stimulates the sebaceous glands, which produces acne," says Murad. And while stress doesn't always surface as acne, it does cause various hormonal changes within your body that ultimately alter the cellular function in your vital organs, all of which affects the appearance of your skin in some form or fashion.

Truth is, we don't need proof of the debilitating effects of stress on our skin by way of acne, as we know all too well what it can do in other ways—among them disrupting our sleep, causing changes in our eating habits, and other practices that we resort to when we fall prey to stress—and *all* of them eventually show up on our skin. So aside from consulting a dermatologist if and when necessary, we do need to do the internal work to fortify and strengthen ourselves so that stress won't manifest itself as a skin condition or concern. Part of so doing lies in making yourself *fit* to fight stress, and I encourage you to review Chapter 5 to see what goes into it. And if you find you need a few ideas for the heart, go back to Chapter 2 and look in on those things that will edify your spirit and put stress in its proper place—beneath you!

However, if you use a milky cleanser to remove your makeup prior to washing your face, be sure to incorporate a toner to check the residue. And if you wear long-wearing eye makeup and lipstick formulas, be sure to use a makeup remover made specifically for these resistant formulas to prevent overhandling these delicate areas, which might cause irritation. Be sure to use loose cotton, which you can purchase by the roll at your local pharmacy or supermarket, to thoroughly remove all traces, as cotton balls don't make the grade! Moisturizers treat and protect the skin as well as trap hydration after cleansing. Finding an appropriate formula, with sunscreen and antioxidants—whether oil-free and noncomedogenic for oily or combination skins, with added humectants for dry skin, or those that are hypoallergenic and fragrance-free for sensitive skin—is doable, thanks to modern-day formulas. Be on the lookout for moisturizers containing state-of-the-art ingredients known as *polyphenols*, powerful antioxidants derived from white grape extract and pomegranate extract that will really improve the quality of your skin while fighting free radicals.

- *Tweak.* To supplement your daily skin care routine between professional facials, experts may recommend applying an at-home mask to rejuvenate, exfoliate, deep-clean, or hydrate skin. You may also need to combine skin care products to address certain concerns. For example, there are times when I tend to break out in my oily zone, primarily on the forehead. To check both the oil and the pimples, I use a blemish control agent in conjunction with my moisturizer in that area. After having a peel, you might need to temporarily use a makeup primer in between your moisturizer and your foundation to keep makeup in place as well as provide a seamless finish while your skin is making a textural adjustment. These and other solutions like them come by way of a knowledgeable expert and by keeping a watchful eye on your skin's behavior.

- *Be good. Don't* squeeze pimples, skip sunscreen, sleep in makeup, use alcohol and products that strip skin, fail to cleanse makeup brushes and sponges weekly, smoke, consume alcoholic beverages, or touch your face unless your hands are scrupulously clean. *Do* change facial towels daily, pillowcases weekly or more frequently if you use styling aids that contain glycerin, mineral oil, or lanolin, use a humidifier in winter, keep hair away from your face, see a dermatologist as needed, or at least yearly, and patch-test all products containing acids.

Ray Watch

Protecting our brown skin from the sun used to be a nonissue. In fact, there was a time when many mothers, mine included, concocted browning oils for their children to enhance our color-rich hues! Many of us also took for granted that the melanin in our skin was a natural defense that kept us out of harm's way when it came to the subject of skin cancer. But times have changed, and despite the fact that melanin does offer us *some* protection, today we recognize the need to shield ourselves on a daily basis as part of a wise care regimen, whether our exposure to the sun's harmful rays is purely incidental or part of a seaside vacation. One serious reality is the fact that skin cancer is now occurring among *us*, and even more disturbing is the fact that it is often undiagnosed, as we don't quite recognize the signs; worse yet, even some experts fail to detect them! The sun's ultraviolet rays cause both premature aging and skin cancer. I can't encourage you enough to visit a dermatologist yearly for a full body exam, and keep a watch on moles or growths, no matter how long you've had them. I've got a mysterious dark bump on one of my legs that I continue to watch, as it has changed its characteristics in the last few years, and since I hate surprises—especially those of an unpleasant nature—I make sure a dermatologist takes a look at it *every* year.

According to Dr. Jeanine B. Downie, director of Image Dermatology in Montclair, New Jersey, malignant melanoma begins as an irregular mole. "I explain to my patients the ABCDs of melanoma: A is for asymmetry of moles, B for irregular borders, C for multiple colors within the mole, and D for large diameter—about the size of a pencil's eraser," she adds. Downie points out that these characteristics call for a skin biopsy, which in turn is interpreted by a specialized skin pathologist. Follow-up treatment is determined by the degree of atypical skin cells and can call for removal or for the mole to be watched closely. Aside from performing your own checks periodically to note any changes, Downie says it's important to recognize that African-Americans, Latinos, and Asians may develop melanomas on the palm of the hands or the soles of the feet, under fingernails and toenails, or in the mouth. So be wise about your exposure to the sun, *period*, not only for these life-altering reasons, but also if you're trying to micromanage uneven pigmentation. The sun activates melanin production, making our efforts at fading dark (hyperpigmented) spots totally in vain.

To protect yourself, wear sunscreen with a sun protection factor (SPF) of at least 15, and preferably one that contains antioxidants, such as vitamins A, C, and E. These two features are easily found in today's tech-savvy products—from lip balms to body lotions—that not only help protect the skin from UV damage but help it to repair itself. I've found that taking this simple precaution really helps me maintain an even tone. Shop for protection according to your needs and desires as well as your skin type. For example, as part of your day-to-day routine, you should be using a light facial moisturizer with sunscreen, one whose texture won't clog pores or disturb your makeup. If your skin falls in the oily or combination categories, perhaps an oil-free gel or balm formulation (lighter and silkier than a lotion) might be more suitable, whereas a lotion would be appropriate for normal to dry skin types. A day at the beach or extended outdoor activities call for a product designed to resist water and sweat, usually a lotion or cream formulation, and a higher SPF, which must still be applied liberally and often. To protect the sensitive, exposed scalp of someone who wears cornrows or flat twists, a gel with an SPF of 30 would fit the bill without any telltale visibility and protect this often-overlooked area from burning. Aside from these considerations, here's what you need to know to make sure you're covered:

- Apply sunscreen daily, at least SPF 15 and at least fifteen minutes before exposure. For those offering broad-spectrum protection by containing a chemical block, such as Parsol 1789 (which protects skin from UVA rays), apply at least thirty minutes in advance. For lengthy exposure, reapply often—every two hours.

- If you use skin care products containing alpha-hydroxy acids or retinol, your skin will be more photosensitive. "Both ingredients make your skin more sensitive to the sun because they exfoliate, taking off the dead skin cells—so you can look fresher or more even," says Downie. So be sure to use an SPF of 30, apply it *before* makeup, and allow time for it to dry thoroughly. And to prevent the ashy cast that many sunscreens have (it comes from the titanium dioxide contained in SPF products that offer this level of protection, and presents a very visible problem for those of us with deeper skin tones), take Downie's advice and incorporate the use of an oil-free moisturizer to help blend and diminish this effect.

- Make sure to use an SPF of at least 15 on the lips, whether you wear lipstick or not, and reapply frequently, as lips don't tan, but they do burn!

- Always avoid the eye area when applying sunscreen products. Instead, look to products made specifically for use on the delicate skin in this area.

- Be sure to use sunscreen even if your cosmetics contain some degree of protection—see the sunscreen in makeup as an added benefit, not a replacement for full protection.

- Avoid sun exposure during the hours of 10:00 A.M. to 4:00 P.M.

Revelations

Forget any notion you might have that facials are a luxury for the pampered set—nothing could be further from the truth. In fact, that's right up there with someone telling you that your car never needs tuning up! Our skin is in a constant state of renewal, shedding dead skin cells every twenty-eight days. As we age, this renewal process slows down. Couple this with the fact that while you're busy living, everything from lack of sleep to the environment, medications, lifestyle, an inadequate diet, and your hormones has its say-so. Include the characteristics of your skin type (whether you're oily, dry, or a combination of both) and your skin's tendencies (enlarged pores, breakouts, lackluster tones, and so on), and know that if you're not getting a professional facial on a monthly basis, your skin isn't in as great a shape as it could be no matter how good it looks. According to Sonya Dakar, of the skin clinic in Los Angeles that bears her name, facials are "important to take impurities out of the skin—i.e., blackheads—because if the skin is clogged, it can develop more breakouts due to the sebaceous glands, which bring oil to the skin." To me, having a facial is like fine-tuning. Having regular oxygen facials has balanced my skin, leaving it even in texture and glowing, and in particular, clarifying my troublesome forehead and erasing my breakouts. Once in a while I have an enzyme peel, which really turns it over, giving me a fresh start. Needless to say, I'm not about to try to force out any blackheads or whiteheads, knowing the risk of injuring my skin and the dark spots that would be sure to follow, so I gladly leave this to a professional, who extracts them during the process of my facial without any negative effects. Then there are those seasonal changes that my skin undergoes—drier and lackluster in winter, oilier and somewhat sensitive in summer. My facialist will adjust the type of mask accordingly and alter my cleansing and moisturizing regimen. Emerging from this treatment with healthy, glowing skin that's as soft as a baby's bottom is only one part of the experience that I love. Caring for my skin as such keeps me from depending on makeup to fake these results, and I can't begin to tell you how much I love the freedom and the confidence this offers me—let alone the ability to do my makeup in minutes! Moreover, like Halle, who also treasures the benefits of regular facials, I really believe in the all-important principle of taking care of what *I* have, first and foremost.

What I've learned from years of talking to the professionals is that a woman's skin changes throughout her lifetime, requiring her to have a real strategy to keep her skin on course and healthy. For model Cynthia Bailey, whose flawless skin heralds the opener to this chapter, it means that a great care regimen is complemented by having regular facials along with her mainstay, a glycolic acid

74

SELF-SEDUCTION

peel, which she affirms gives her new skin. The busy model, whose long days on assignment are spent under the glare of hot studio lights in a full face of makeup, attributes this precise care more to the changes in her skin since the birth of her daughter Noelle. "It's gone from no maintenance to low maintenance," she proclaims. Bailey says that pre-baby, she could go to bed in makeup, but now those days are gone. "I have to look after it a bit more—I need to exfoliate a lot, every two days if not every night," and she uses a facial moisturizer with sunscreen. For singer and actress Erykah Badu, clay facials and mud baths are a beauty priority second only to nutrition. And actress LaTanya Richardson Jackson relies on customized facials once or twice a month to help maintain her lush chocolate complexion, which is blemish-free. She too cites changes in her life that call for sound care habits: "My skin's constantly changing. It used to be very plump and buoyant. I'm finding that now it doesn't want to take a lot and requires that I be easy with it." Richardson Jackson, who finds herself paying attention ever more closely to her skin, says she knows she can't go out without sunscreen. "Halfway through the day, I feel tight and wrinkly and my skin is saying, 'Protect me.'" Actress and singer Vanessa Williams, for whom acne has been a challenge since her teen years, says now she has to work a little differently at keeping her skin clear. "One of my concerns is as I get older, my skin is getting drier," she says. As a solution, Williams, who says she's tried everything from tetracycline to Accutane as well as fruit acids, found her adult acne called for a different strategy, one that is gentle, topical, and nondrying, and is inclusive in the facials she says she loves to get.

Skin truths like these hold fast for many of us, no matter what our profession. Keeping a demanding schedule, compounded by long hours, perhaps air travel, occasional missteps (like sleeping in makeup or improper product usage, even self-diagnosis of our skin and its needs), life changes such as giving birth or menopause, and certainly the changes we incur as we age—all these are factors that cause our skin to behave differently, and all can be helped by having consistent professional care that's discerning. Many sisters in the know schedule their monthly facials around their menstrual cycle, particularly at the time when breakouts are most likely to occur; others schedule it as a form of routine maintenance. They have resolved that a healthy complexion, just like any other aspect of their beauty, requires specific attention.

When you have a professional facial, it should always begin with a consultation. Since you know your skin's behavior better than anyone else, this is the time to give the aesthetician an honest assessment of it. Tell her also about any sensitivity you're aware of and any medications you're on, and inform her of your care routine. Your skin will then be analyzed to determine its condition. After that, just close your eyes, relax, and prepare to be treated. During the facial a massage is given to stimulate circulation and loosen up any imbedded toxins in your pores, under a mist of comfortably hot steam. Variations on this part of the process may occur as needed, depending on your skin type or its condition. Cornelia Zircu, aesthetician at the Peninsula Spa in New York City, offers this example: "If a person has problem skin, massage is a no-no, as it produces more oil." The facial continues with a gentle exfoliation and any necessary extractions performed manually; this is followed by a mask suitable for your complexion and its needs, such as a purifying clay-based mask, which further exfoliates and absorbs skin debris and oil, for oily or combination skin, or a hydrating mask, many of which contain mineral water, lipids, and other ingredients to help bind moisture to dry, parched skin.

Also in the skin-refining category are those technological wonders otherwise known as chemical peels, which rejuvenate your complexion by means of exfoliating the top layer of dead cells and stimulating cellular renewal. These are best performed by a dermatologist or aesthetician who knows his or her stuff when it comes to our skin. The process begins with an evaluation of your skin to determine your needs and the ideal chemical to achieve the results. Many experts will do a patch test to check for any sensitivities you might have. Once the analysis has been made and the results of the patch test have given an all-clear, your skin will be cleansed in preparation for the peel. The typical process begins with the application of a solution containing the appropriate acid—alpha-hydroxy, beta-hydroxy, or trichloroacetic—to exfoliate the skin. During the course of the procedure you may experience a slight burning or prickling sensation, which may last after the process is completed. Beyond this, you may find your skin to be sensitive for twenty-four to seventy-two hours after being treated, so, needless to say, it's best not to have this done prior to a big event. There are also *enzyme peels*, based on natural ingredients—pumpkin, papaya, sage, chamomile, and the like—that will give you the benefits of exfoliation with less or no irritation. "Enzymes are very smart in that they don't digest *live* cells, only dead cells," says Zircu. She and other experts such as Dakar favor these mild, natural peels for women of color.

The mildest acids commonly used in chemical peels are *alpha-hydroxy acids* (AHAs), such as lactic or glycolic acid. These exfoliate, lighten discolorations, improve dullness, soften and smooth the skin, and lessen the appearance of fine lines. *Beta-hydroxy acids* (BHAs), such as salicylic acid, are another alternative. Unlike AHAs, beta-hydroxy acids are self-neutralizing, meaning that they don't require an additional solution to halt their action. According to Dr. Cheryl Burgess, of the Center for Dermatology, in Washington, D.C., they address "anything that has to do with your pores, such as acne." Some have found them to also be helpful for pimples as well as blackheads. Another type of peel that also addresses acne is a *vitamin A* or *retinoic acid* peel. "If you had to choose any vitamin that was beneficial for problem or acne-prone skin, it would be vitamin A," adds Burgess. Then there's *trichloroacetic acid* (TCA), which is used for a medium-depth peel. It penetrates the skin at a level that facilitates collagen renewal, reduces fine lines, and decreases the appearance of large pores and moderate acne scarring. This type of peel should always be done by a medical professional and at the lowest strength, as it causes skin to peel and carries the risk of additional scarring for those with deeper skin tones. When considering any peel, be advised that most experts recommend only the mildest formulas for women of color, and strongly urge us to shun those that contain phenol. "This type of peel lightens the skin, so African-Americans should avoid it, as it can be permanent. It also can cause cardiac arrhythmias; therefore it is a procedure that is done under cardiac monitoring," says Burgess. Despite the safety of most peels, for those of us with darker skin tones, there is still a greater risk of discoloration. Be sure to discuss all your options with a pro you trust, so that together you can make the wisest choice.

Another refining process that can lead to smoother skin, improve texture irregularities, and reduce fine lines is microdermabrasion (not to be confused with dermabrasion, an older procedure that can cause color changes). This procedure, where a gentle spray of aluminum oxide crystals is administered to the face and then lightly sucked away along with dead skin cells, is also performed by both dermatologists and aestheticians. According to Burgess, it's a procedure that's ideal for someone with acne scarring, deep pits, and surface irregularities. It's worth noting that the procedure you'll receive in a doctor's office will differ from that available in a salon or spa due to the fact that the machines offered to doctors have more intense settings than those offered to aestheticians. "With the physician's systems, I can do scar revision," adds Burgess. On the other hand, those sold to salons and spas, says Dr. Robin Ashinoff, chief of dermatological surgery and laser at New York University Medical Center and chief of cosmetic dermatology at Hackensack Medical Center in Hackensack, New Jersey, "don't abrade the skin very deeply." And still I say, for those of us on the deeper end of the color spectrum, take care when selecting an expert to refine your skin in this manner. In the hands of an overzealous person, hyperpigmentation is very possible—to me that's not a great trade-off for minimized pores! I learned several years ago that there is no rhyme or reason to the way melanin rushes in when our skin is injured or assaulted. For example, your sister friend who's of a caramel hue will more than likely spend less time fading a dark spot left behind by a healing mosquito bite or a cystic bump than you will if your skin tone is like mine, so find a knowledgeable expert for whom this is a specialty if you're looking to diminish acne scarring.

Whether you're looking to deep-clean, minimize breakouts, or boost radiance, there's an effective facial process to help you get there. Remember that although treatments and their names and ingredients will vary, most aestheticians will pretty much follow the basics:

- Cleansing

- Exfoliating

- Extraction of impurities

- Application of a suitable mask

- Moisturization to complete the process

But before you pick up the phone to book any treatment, don't self-diagnose. Just because a facial sounds good doesn't make it right for you. It's best to schedule an hour with an aesthetician and allow her to make the call about what type of facial your skin needs. A good facialist will do this anyway, no matter what the client has booked, as she'll want what's best for her client's skin. Zircu reminds us that we wouldn't tell a doctor what we need; instead we would allow him or her to make the determination. Keep in mind that a good aesthetician will customize your treatment based on your skin's condition. Having said as much, here then is a checklist of those facials that give us the most mileage when properly matched to skin type and its needs and when combined with an appropriate at-home care regimen:

Deep-cleansing/purifying. A basic treatment suitable for most skin types, but especially beneficial for those with oily/combination skin. It removes impurities and nourishes the skin, leaving it soft and smooth.

Oxygen. For all skin types, but especially revitalizes dull, dehydrated skin with the addition of pure oxygen to nourish the cells, increase collagen production, and bring about a glow.

Vitamin C. A powerful antioxidant that removes dead skin cells, imparts brightness, and creates radiant new skin—an instantly de-aging boost for all skin types!

Hydrating. Aimed at nurturing dry or mature skin or skin dehydrated by environmental factors, this treatment stimulates circulation, softens, and replenishes moisture.

Refining. Usually involves the addition of alpha- or beta-hydroxy acids to enhance exfoliation, soften, and renew the skin.

As with all treatments or products containing acids, you have to find your match in order to achieve the beautifying benefits, so it's best to have a patch test or inform the aesthetician of any known sensitivity. I've seen an AHA facial burn our skin (evidenced by a dark mark), and no matter how temporary this is, that's a problem. So regardless of how gentle the expert tells you the ingredients are, if she's treating you for the first time or if this is your first experience with this kind of facial, insist on a patch test or ask for an alternative. And if you've begun having these treatments but find that your skin is irritated or remains too shiny in spots, talk to your expert about cutting back, going for a milder solution, or another option.

Undercover: Support Strategies for Special Concerns

In my mind-set as an editor, it's always about sharing *the* solution to a problem. What I'm finding more and more as a woman is that it isn't always that simple. Although many of us have similar skin care concerns or trouble zones, our solutions can vary depending on the cause and our unique makeup. This is why consulting an expert to achieve your desires should always be your first approach, as the given remedy will usually need to be customized for your skin. I don't want you to analyze your skin any more than I would analyze mine; the risk of damage is too great. I'd rather help you by telling you those truths you can use. Take acne, for example—according to Zircu, who travels the nation teaching aestheticians, the condition has a number of triggers, and in turn it's treated in many ways. Sally Pansing Kravich, CNHP, a natural health consultant and iridologist with a bicoastal practice in Los Angeles and New York, offers this example: "If a person has acne and, say, they have a congested lymphatic system and a congested colon, I'd get them on a diet that wouldn't have any fried foods and insoluble fats in it. And since their lymph is congested, they'd need to sweat and drink a lot of water, cut out any kind of sodas whatsoever, cut out wheat and any white-flour products, and probably do a bowel cleaner. I would follow this up with a blood purifier and builder such as chlorophyll, as when you clean the blood you automatically clean the lymph. So there's an internal cleansing as well as a cleanup of the blood," concludes Kravich. As you can see, clearing up certain skin conditions can call for a multi-pronged approach. In truth, it's usually better to address skin concerns from both within and without, as this is really the wise way to invest in yourself. Again, know the skin *you're* in.

On the other hand, great strides have been made in the area of skin care. Many are more suitable for Caucasians than for those of us with melanin-rich skin, but I nevertheless want you to be aware of them!so that you can be informed and empowered. Many times your expert will recommend over-the-counter products or advise their use in combination with those that are available only by prescription or of a cosmeceutical nature. Some of the treatments described in the "Revelations" section may be appropriate as well. Here are some guidelines that the experts rely on when treating our common concerns.

PIMPLES These fine bumps can be hormonal (arising prior to menstruation) or result from overactive sebaceous glands, aggressive products, hair preparations, too much sun exposure, exercising in makeup, heavy moisturizers, or skin care products containing fragrance. *Treatment:* Experts will conduct a profile to determine possible causes and advise on product usage and care habits. Depending on how sensitive your skin is, you may be counseled to try over-the-counter products containing salicylic acid, mild sulfur, or benzoyl peroxide. Alternatively, you may be recommended cosmeceuticals, or oral or topical antibiotics may be prescribed.

BLACKHEADS AND WHITEHEADS Blockages of the oil glands, with blackheads resembling clogged pores (contrary to popular belief, they are clogged not with dirt but with debris from the skin and bacteria) and whiteheads resembling medium to fine pimples capped with a small white ball. *Treatment:* Deep-cleansing facials, product regimes, or preparations that may include salicylic acid, retinoids, or benzoyl peroxide.

FLESH MOLES Otherwise known as *dermatosis papulosa nigra*, which can occur all over the face and upper body. They are increasingly common with age and are hereditary. *Treatment:* Moles are removed through a process known as electro-desiccation, in which they are lightly burned or seared. This treatment causes them to fall off without scarring; however, there is a risk of temporary discoloration. They can also be frozen using liquid nitrogen and allowed to fall off.

EXCESSIVE OILINESS A hormonal or stress-related problem. *Treatment:* There's nothing that can control your oil glands; however, salicylic acid and benzoyl peroxide are usually prescribed to help reduce the oil. Over-the-counter mattifying products can also be used in conjunction to keep oil from disturbing makeup.

RESISTANT HYPERPIGMENTATION Excessive production of melanin that can result from sun exposure, birth control pills, estrogen, inflammation from acne, insect bites, or any other trauma to the skin. *Treatment:* In some cases hyperpigmentation will fade on its own, with the exception of when it occurs in areas where there's friction, such as on the elbows or the knees, or is the result of deep or repeated trauma. Experts will usually assess the area to determine whether discoloration is limited to the epidermis or extends into the skin's dermis layer. Depending on the assessment, which determines the type of treatment used to address it as well as the duration, hydroquinone in its over-the-counter strength (2 percent) or in prescription strength (3–4 percent) will be used to fade the area; teaming hydroquinone with alpha- and beta-hydroxy acids or with a glycolic chemical peel will help speed up the process. "If the mark is from a burn, however, there are other factors involved, such as scar tissue," says Burgess. In this case, a dermatologist may elect to treat it with a laser, such as the Q-switched or Lyra laser, to break it up. Glycolic acid in a superficial peel will also address resistant hyperpigmentation on elbows and knees, as will treating them with the Q-switched laser.

Knowing when to incorporate the help of an aesthetician or a dermatologist in caring for your skin can be confusing at times. But I agree with Dr. Howard Murad, assistant professor of dermatology at UCLA, who suggests that you ask yourself, "How can I take care of my skin?" and do so before you have a problem. If you have a specific complaint about your skin, hair, or nails or a persistent condition such as acne, it's best to begin by seeing a dermatologist. Likewise, be sure to consult with a dermatologist for repeated breakouts or anything that raises a question like, say, the mysterious growth on my leg that I mentioned earlier. Always be sure to schedule an appointment sooner rather than later because patience *isn't* a virtue, particularly when there's cause for concern. More often than not, the longer you wait to have it checked out, the more damage control will be required, and it can also lessen your chances of optimal results. According to Ashinoff, it's also best to look to a dermatologist when considering certain types of procedures, such as Botox—a medical procedure that relaxes deep creases on the forehead and between the eyes for up to four months through injections of botulinum toxin. "This has risks and benefits, so it's important to be in a medical setting—if you have a problem or a question, there's someone on call twenty-four hours a day. *That* you would not get through a spa."

It's best to see an aesthetician for facials or superficial light peels, skin-conditioning body treatments, and recommendations on skin care products, providing you needn't be under a doctor's care for a particular condition. I also like seeing an aesthetician occasionally for microdermabrasion on my feet. To me it's a great head start to sandal-ready feet. However, when it comes to dermatologists and aestheticians, it's really not a question of either/or—both should be a part of that temple management team I mentioned earlier that keeps you at your best. So for me, there are concerns that I watch or care for under the guidance of a dermatologist and those that I care for through the advice and services of an aesthetician. Since I don't have a condition that requires routine dermatological care, I'm seeing the aesthetician more frequently. She's the one who helps to repair my skin from the dehydrating effects of air travel, analyze any changes, or recommend product additions or subtractions. She also pampers my emotional beauty through her nurturing treatments and gentle guidance, and that's a plus I wouldn't want to be without. Burgess, whose staff includes aestheticians, says physicians and aestheticians complement each other by working hand in hand. "If someone has acne, they'll see me first, and perhaps I'll put them on cosmeceuticals—not prescription or over-the-counter products, but nevertheless of the caliber that can only be dispensed by a dermatologist." (More and more you'll also find that a number of dermatologists have their own skin care lines.) "The aesthetician will go over specifically what they're supposed to do, and if I need the patient steamed or deep-cleaned, again that's when my aesthetician will come into play." At the Beyond Spa in Hackensack, New Jersey, aestheticians also perform follow-up care from deeper peels performed by doctors such as Ashinoff once the patient is completely healed. So again, it's about consulting the right experts for the care of your skin and any procedures you may require or simply be interested in.

To find a dermatologist in your area, contact the National Medical Association (NMA), an organization that promotes the interests of physicians and patients of African descent, at 1-888-662-7497, where a live operator will help you locate physicians by specialty or by location.

ECZEMA Inflammation of the skin that leads to persistent itching and possibly cracked skin, rashes, or bacterial and viral skin infections; often triggered by stress. *Treatment:* Avoid harsh soap, detergents, woolens, and any other known skin irritants. Oil baths and steroid creams and ointments may be helpful. Newer still are topical immunomodulators, which help symptoms by inhibiting the over-reaction of T cells, which provokes skin inflammation. The use of a humidifier is also helpful.

Skin Truths: Ages 20–50+

Growing up, I was on fast-forward—I couldn't wait to be an adult. In fact, many of my elders used to say, "Child, don't be in such a hurry to be grown before your time—you've got all your life to be grown." Little did I know the truth of that, especially as it applied to what to expect when it came to life, let alone my skin. Addressing changes that seemingly arrived with every big birthday would have been a heck of a navigation process had I not been exposed, in my role as an editor, to every new product or ingredient the beauty industry had to offer, as well as a host of experts starting when I was twenty-five. Having firsthand knowledge has made the process of making adjustments here and there a smooth ride.

Genetics and the way we age in general have undoubtedly made a significant contribution to the skin we're in. In fact, when I look at today's baby-boomers in their forties and fifties, their faces and temples (not to mention their lives) easily mimic those of women in their thirties and forties! Why, I get a kick every time I hear Star Jones, who has the most fabulous nerve, get on television and tell the nation, "Black don't crack!"

"African-American women age much later on than Caucasian women—they can see fine lines and wrinkles at twenty or thirty, but it's very unusual for our skin to display fine lines and wrinkling at that age. What we see commonly is uneven pigmentation, light or dark blotches, and I think that's probably a function of sun exposure," says Dr. Taylor. In my presentations to beauty companies I get a particular joy out of telling folks that by the time we wrinkle, "those divas have earned the right," and you'd be hard pressed to find any one of them trying to diminish those signs of experience. Seriously, though, you know that's just not how we measure our beauty. Nevertheless, there are some strategies that we need to be aware of that can and do play a role in how lovely our skin is as well as things we need to know about that can cause us to age in our own unique ways before our time or that can compromise our skin's integrity. Times have changed, and there are things that cause us to manage our skin differently than our elders—from the nature of the foods we eat and the lives we live to the fact

Model Tia Holland

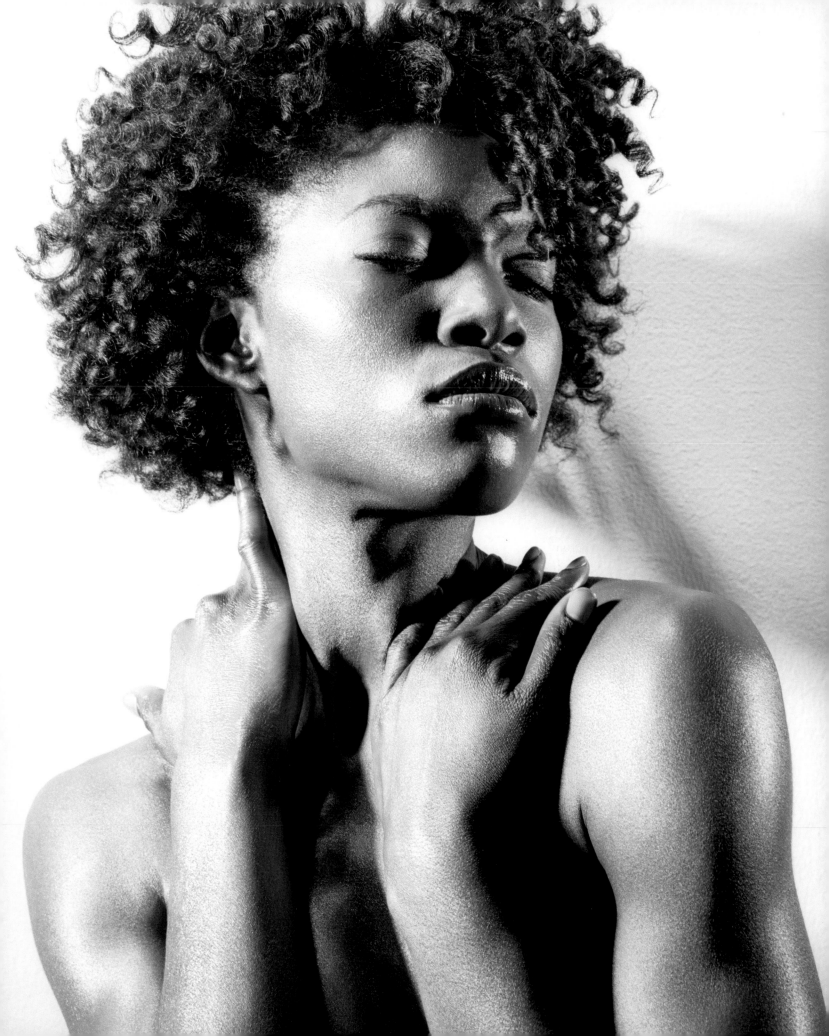

that the ozone layer is quite different than it was back in the day. According to Dr. Murad, it's really a question of what age your skin is. And there are a litany of things that age skin, including stress, pollution, smog, sun, poor diet, et cetera, et cetera, all of which have one thing in common: free-radical damage. So while many of our elders may have had glorious skin with a soap-and-water regimen, we have to think and do differently because this is not true for us now, nor of our future. Here's what you should know at a glance about the skin you're in and its journey.

YOUR TWENTIES Even though skin during this decade is plump and in a state of optimal renewal, now is a time for consistent prevention. During your twenties a lot of unseen damage is occurring. According to Murad, everything from the lifestyle habits we take for granted (activities that keep us awake longer) to attending parties where there's smoke and alcohol and other things that pollute the skin is causing damage. He says, "An ounce of prevention is worth a pound of cure." Establishing a skin care regimen that includes a moisturizer with antioxidants (vitamins A, C, and E) as well as taking them internally is key. If breakouts or acne is a concern, it's important to consult a dermatologist to prevent exacerbation or scarring. This is also a time to pay attention to healthful eating and to form other good habits such as having monthly facials, getting enough sleep, and being good to your skin overall, as outlined in "Conscious Care." Know too that everything from yo-yo dieting to birth-control pills has an effect on the skin. The former causes it to lose elasticity, while the latter, even though it may clear up acne, has been associated with melasma (brown pigmentation on the cheeks, around the eyes, and sometimes on the forehead or above the lips; it is also associated with the hormonal changes of pregnancy), so using a broad-spectrum sunscreen as well as a gentle fade product is important.

YOUR THIRTIES Minimal signs of aging can appear, even though we don't attribute them to age, because they don't materialize as things we associate with age on women of other cultures, such as fine lines. At this stage flesh moles may begin to appear. Melasma can also be a concern. Cell turnover begins to slow down, and overall unevenness may be more prevalent. Dr. Taylor advises thinking about glycolic acid products to help exfoliate in a gentle fashion; others address these concerns with hydroquinone or a mild but effective botanically based bleaching agent such as kojic acid, licorice extract, or bearberry extract (which, according to Murad, minimizes discoloration). Aside from these factors, acne may show up for the first time; Murad points out that it can be stress-related, calling for specific treatment that will address it without drying out your skin overall. Hyperpigmentation that is a reaction to inflammation, such as with acne, can also occur. "When there's inflammation from a pimple, it stimulates the melanocytes to produce melanin," Murad says. If you're of a deeper hue, your melanin is more active than that of somebody who has fairer skin, and so when the skin inflammation disappears, you may be left with a spot. This is treatable with preparations that include any of the ingredients mentioned, but make sure to apply the product to the dark spots *only*. In your thirties, your care regimen may need to take into account your skin's need for more moisture. Don't miss out on the benefits of antioxidants, both in topical preparations and taken as supplements. Your skin can receive a much-needed boost from monthly facials. And don't forget the protection afforded by sunscreen.

YOUR FORTIES Your skin may have become drier and a little less radiant, acne is a thing of the past, and if enlarged pores were a problem, they are less visible now. Declining levels of estrogen, which maintain collagen and elastin, may begin to show up as a slight lack of firmness. Some women may experience early menopause, which may result in increased facial hair, a loss of scalp hair, and a renewed concern with acne because of the lack of estrogen to prevent sebaceous activity. Your skin care regimen may include products containing such noteworthy ingredients as copper, said to stimulate collagen production and increase hydration, or vitamin C, which promotes radiance. You may also decide to have any flesh moles removed. Look to oxygen facials or superficial chemical peels, advises Taylor, as part of your routine for skin that glows. If facial hair is a concern, consulting an electrologist is an option.

YOUR FIFTIES AND BEYOND The onset of menopause will bring about a reduction in estrogen and collagen production. A slight loss of firmness may occur, along with fine lines under the eyes. Women of lighter skin tones in their fifties and sixties, according to Taylor, will see fine wrinkling, further discoloration, and sagging. Sebaceous glands secrete less oil, and so skin is drier. A nurturing regimen to specifically address the needs of women in this phase is a great solution, as are nourishing facials and increased support of the skin through nutritional advice and supplements containing B vitamins, antioxidants, and amino acids.

Supple Gestures

I am more than convinced that my skin looks its best in summer. Therefore, I decided a long time ago that I was going to do everything in my power to keep it looking that great year round. When you think about it, our bodies positively glow during the warmer months (year round for those of you who live in subtrop-

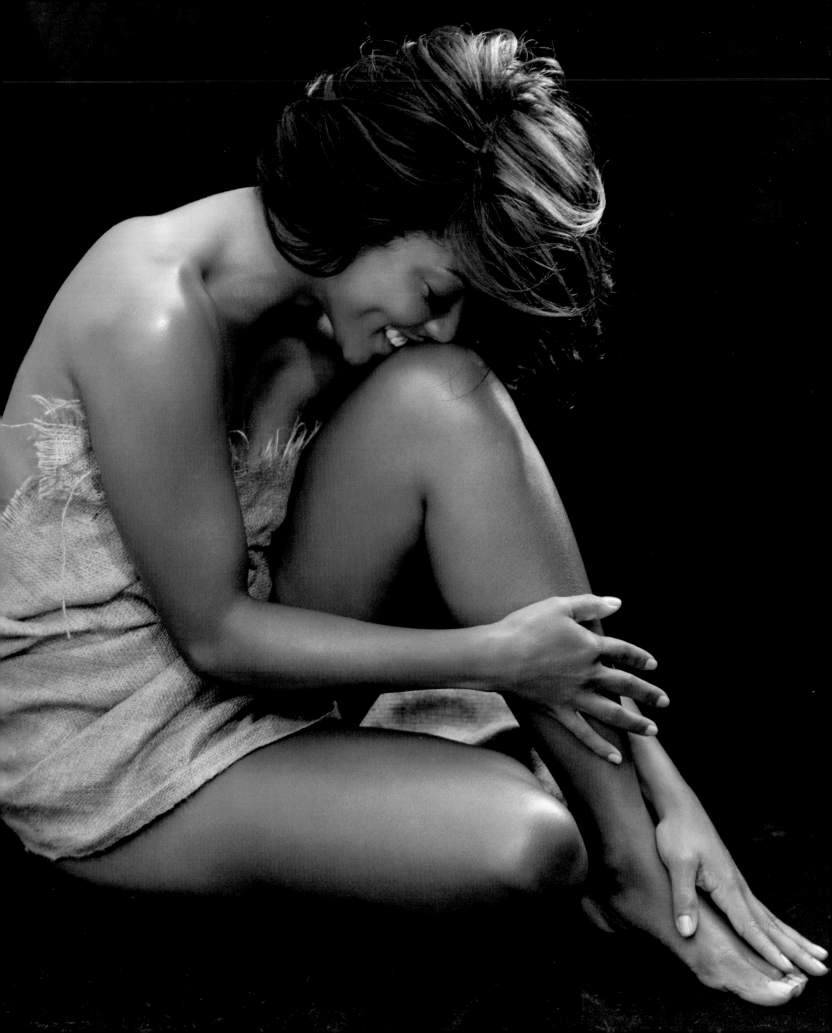

ical climates)—why, even those persistent dry areas seem to behave with minimal attention. Well, the real lowdown here is humidity—in other words, moisture.

Believe it or not, the key to smooth, hydrated skin that won't turn ashy when you least expect it lies in exfoliating dead cells on a weekly basis. Incorporating a good salt- or sugar-based body scrub is nonirritating and reveals nice healthy skin that will better hold on to moisture. Apply the scrub to dry, not wet, skin for the most effective results. Alternatively, use a loofah on a weekly basis while bathing. With either a scrub or a loofah, follow up with a hydrating shower gel so that skin won't come squeaky clean—a real no-no! After bath or shower, apply a massage oil in conjunction with your body lotion or cream, or use a dry-oil spray first. Trust me, this combination really seals your efforts.

Shea butter, which comes from the cradle of civilization (and is not to be confused with cocoa butter, which is too greasy), is unsurpassed as a hydrator in my book. For unevenness, incorporate the use of a body moisturizer with vitamin C or AHAs. I also like the use of a body serum with retinol, as I find it really retexturizes the skin, making it appear smooth and compact. And come spring, when you're ready to step out without hose but your legs aren't there yet, self-tanners are a real boon. Back facials are a terrific boost for those prone to break-outs, as are some of today's high-tech skin care lines that feature clay masks or sprays with ingredients such as salicylic acid or retinol that can be applied at home with the help of a sister friend or spouse.

Pampering spa treats such as paraffin-mud and seaweed wraps also treat dry body skin, leaving it soft and glowing. In fact, TLC and extra attention go a long way, period. One would never know that actress Garcelle Beauvais-Nilon, of ABC's *NYPD Blue*, works at keeping eczema at bay by putting a particular emphasis on moisturizing her skin, or that model Wendy Brooks suffered with eczema when she was growing up. Brooks attributes her parents' care, in particular that of her dad, for the way her skin appears today. Says Brooks of his care of her and her sister, who also had this condition, "My father was the one who bathed all of us, and then creamed us with an intensive lotion and our prescription—like a cortisone cream—only on those areas. This was a religious routine morning and night." She believes that it's due to his faithfulness that she grew out of it. "When I look at my skin I can't believe I had eczema. I had white blotches on my face and rough, rough skin that was very itchy. When we would go to hot climates (we grew up in Canada), our skin would itch, so he made us sleep with gloves on so we wouldn't scratch," she adds.

Model Wendy Brooks

Tackling Cellulite

Cellulite—that bumpy, dimpled fat that commonly appears on our buttocks, hips, thighs, and abdomens—does not discriminate, affecting women of all ages, shapes, and sizes. In truth, there aren't many of us who get through life without it, as it's both hormonal and genetic, which explains why even thin women get it. And contrary to what you might hear at many spas about toxins and impurities, there's no scientific evidence that cellulite is anything other than regular fat. Therein lies the good news, because that means you have a real opportunity to eliminate it or at least bring about an improvement.

Here's how you take action:

Start moving A consistent routine that includes cardiovascular exercise—jogging, cycling, or swimming—for thirty minutes at least three times a week (to burn calories and improve your circulation) and weight training (to work your major muscles *intensively)* are your best hope for firming and smoothing your skin's appearance. Exercise is said to reduce the size of the fat cells, and it definitely tones up loose skin, making cellulite less visible. According to Gary Liggins of the S.W.A.T.T. Fitness Camp in West Hollywood, California, you want to target those areas that seem to be cellulite-prone by shaping them with core exercises that work the abs, the lower back, and the glutes in conjunction with squats, lunges, and leg presses, all of which, says Liggins, "will help tremendously." And, adds Liggins's stacked wife, Valerie, who's part of the team of trainers that work out such celeb sisters as Cookie Johnson and LaTanya Richardson Jackson, "when you have less muscle, all you have is fat there, and yes, that reveals cellulite." Now, this is not to suggest that you can spot-train. It simply means that as part of an overall workout regime that includes some type of cardiovascular exercise, you will up the ante on the exercises that shape and define your muscles. The key is to get a personal trainer or find a class where the instructor really understands how to assist you with the proper exercises that'll help you reach your goals. At S.W.A.T.T., which is a four-week, five-days-a-week program, those dolls are taking to the beach or hitting the mountains as part of their daily "boot camp," like Marines—and mind you, going beyond their original goals! Michelle Adams, a certified personal trainer and fitness instructor at New York City's Equinox Gyms, assists her clients in their efforts with aerobic workouts, African dance, kick-boxing, and strength training with lighter weights (focusing on the lower body with increased repetitions) and by going back to the old-school days of calisthenics in many of her sessions. Her goal is to include a medley of different exercises so that the body doesn't get used to the strength-training routine.

According to Adams, these are the things that change the game by altering the proportion of body fat to muscle mass and giving you a smoother, firmer appearance. "It's really a matter of the subcutaneous fat cells getting smaller," she says, "and when that happens, you start to see less and less cellulite."

MODIFY YOUR DIET For certain, cutting out sweets, eating less fat, and increasing your intake of fresh fruits and vegetables will enhance your efforts. So will getting enough water—ideally one and a half to two liters a day. And be sure to increase your water intake even more if you drink coffee, caffeinated beverages, or alcohol, all of which are dehydrating. According to the experts, when you're dehydrated, your body holds on to more fluid, making you look puffy, thus exacerbating the appearance of cellulite—and that's the last thing you need! Try to stay on the natural path; processed foods and those laden with chemicals and dyes are a real no-no for your glorious temple. Your organs have enough work to do without trying to process these additives.

SUPERSIZE YOUR EFFORTS Coupling the use of topical retinoids, which can make skin appear smoother, with a modified diet and consistent exercise offers you a more effective program to address cellulite. According to Beverly Hills plastic surgeon Dr. John A. Grossman, "skin creams with retinoids and alpha- and beta-hydroxy acids, through promoting exfoliation, will help keep the skin cells plump and, by the reaction to them, activate new collagen." Grossman suggests trying over-the-counter formulas that contain these ingredients, albeit at a minimal level at first because of the irritation associated with stronger formulas, and then building up to prescription strength. Many experts also believe in the benefits of Endermologie (a mechanical treatment that manipulates and massages the skin, much like a deep-tissue massage, with the aim of breaking down fat and improving circulation and lymphatic drainage). It is said to be the most effective method for reducing the appearance of cellulite. To see results, you must be willing to commit to as many as ten to twenty sessions initially, at an average cost of $100 to $150 each, and then follow-up visits once or twice a month thereafter. Keep in mind that Endermologie is most suitable for those who are close to their ideal weight. And while there are many women who have tried this approach with satisfactory results, the American Society of Plastic Surgeons and the American Society for Aesthetic Plastic Surgery have published a number of articles documenting scientific studies that were done on this practice and found it to be *ineffective*. For more information about this procedure, call the LPG Group—the creator of the original subcutaneous technology: 1-800-222-3911; or log on to www.endermologie.com.

In the meantime, pamper yourself and reward your efforts with the use of one of the topical creams described above to aid in smoothing out the skin; if you find them irritating, try a body scrub and a good cellulite product. Most of them contain caffeine, which is said to reduce water in the skin and make it appear firmer, however temporary the results. You should be aware that they have absolutely no effect whatsoever on the fatty deposits themselves, but hey, who's checking? What you care about most, even while playing the waiting game, is the appearance of smooth skin, and some of these products do provide that while they are on the skin. Going for a professional massage—particularly a deep-tissue massage or lymphatic drainage—will temporarily complement your efforts as well. Know, however, that liposuction (an invasive procedure that gets rid of unwanted fat) is not an option, as it cannot correct cellulite. Most of all, recognize that you're not going to be able to reverse genetics, but Grossman points out that for most of us, what we see when it comes to cellulite is 70 percent genetic and 30 percent environmental. "It's the things that we choose to do that make the difference," he says, "those things that harm the tissues—like sun exposure that results in a deep tan, because that promotes fracturing of the elastic fibers and loosening of that skin before its time. If you change that thirty percent, you can ultimately make a difference." Other factors such as maintaining your weight and eating a healthy diet—again, combined with proper exercise—also play a significant role.

I know that when I combined Tae Bo with biking three times a week, weight training, and a commitment to the right foods, I was able to step into a two-piece bathing suit with confidence for the first time since I was a teenager! So I'm here to tell you that diligence and hard work can pay off. However, if you should find that your best efforts don't eliminate cellulite entirely, don't trip it. What you will have gained in the process is a stronger, leaner, and healthier body, and that, my sisters, is something to pat yourselves on the back about!

Vein Glory

Like you, I so hate a beauty concern that cramps my style. Take spider or varicose veins. To this day many a sister with a great pair of legs never hits the beach or steps out of a pair of trousers because of these esteem breakers. Oftentimes genetics are to blame, but so too are a woman's hormones, birth control pills, estrogen replacement, and other contributing factors, among them weight gain, a sedentary lifestyle, high heels, crossing your legs, and spending extensive periods on your feet.

Despite these factors, this is another area where women of color can have the victory due to technological advances designed specifically to get rid of them. One such option for those with spider veins is *sclerotherapy*, in which doctors inject a saline or detergent solution into the veins that causes them to collapse and disappear. Another, newer option is *laser surgery* with the new YAG laser (also great for veins that are so tiny that they cannot be treated by sclerotherapy); unlike previous lasers, which could result in pigmentary problems for darker skin tones, the YAG laser goes deeper into skin, bypassing the layer that holds pigment, and destroys the vein. For varicose veins there's also the *closure technique*, where a small catheter is inserted into a small incision behind the knee and guided by doppler ultrasound. The catheter contains an electrode that emits energy inside the vein, causing it to heat, collapse, and seal shut. Both procedures are performed in the office by a medical doctor. With sclerotherapy, no anesthesia is necessary, as there is only minimal discomfort associated with this technique, such as the pricking sensation of the needle, and a possible burning sensation when the solution is initially injected. With the laser, the discomfort is also minimal, no more than the kind of sensation that would accompany the sting of a rubber band when snapped against the skin each time the pulse is administered.

Following sclerotherapy, you will be advised not to work out for twenty-four hours, and after laser surgery not to physically exert yourself or take baths for three days, although you can return to work right away after both procedures. After these treatments, women are advised to wear prescribed support hose to maintain pressure on the veins. Treating spider veins with sclerotherapy can require three to six sessions. The downsides to these treatments include some bruising and possibly some swelling. Occasionally after sclerotherapy, small clots can form at the point of the injections; however, they can easily be removed by your doctor. For people of color, any type of laser therapy can cause discoloration, in this case either lightening or darkening of the skin where it is utilized, so be sure to discuss this risk with your doctor before scheduling this procedure.

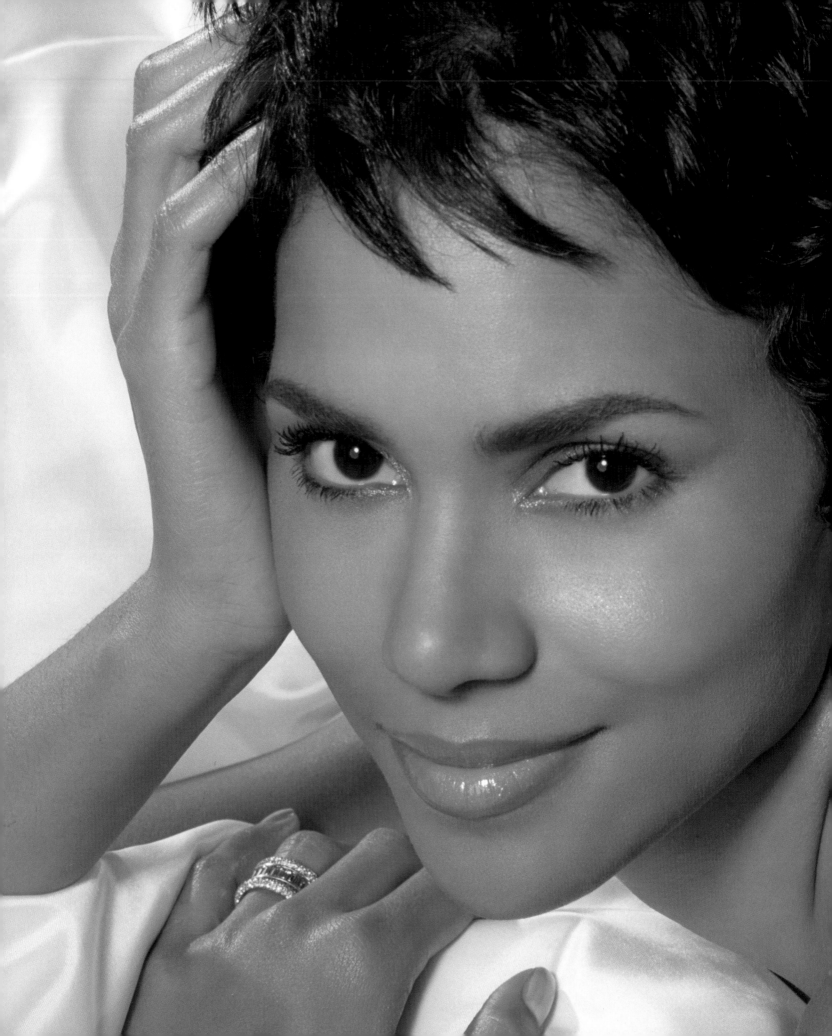

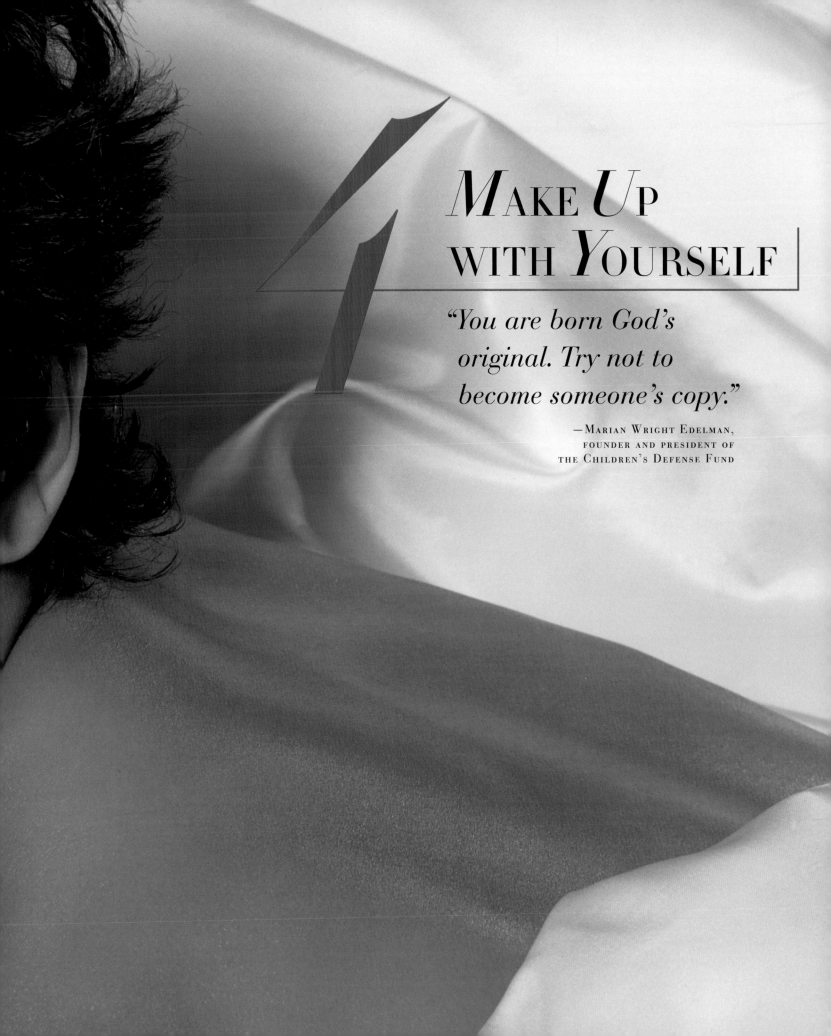

MAKE UP WITH YOURSELF

"You are born God's original. Try not to become someone's copy."

—MARIAN WRIGHT EDELMAN,
FOUNDER AND PRESIDENT OF
THE CHILDREN'S DEFENSE FUND

I f there's one thing I'm absolutely fascinated about, it's makeup. To me it's a form of eye candy, and every new shadow, liner, lipstick—you name it— makes my heart race just a little bit more than the one I fell in love with yester- day! Ever since I was a child, I lived for the moment to explore the many possibilities in beauty, and I can tell you makeup was and still is chief. Perhaps it's because I love to indulge what some would call a big imagination, or maybe it's because my mother, who was a professional makeup artist, always took it to the next level. She was also quite a makeup maven personally. Why, she could serve a pair of brows and pencil in a beauty mark that would make my father's heart forget to beat. She was passionate about makeup and shopped for it with a keen eye that always delivered the best finds. She would come home from her trips to Europe with Sarah Vaughan with the most incredible goodies, such as foundation that matched her brown skin perfectly and came in the most sensual miniature bottles. Back then I never wondered why she had to cross the Atlantic to find them—I just knew I wanted some! I didn't put two and two together, as they say, until much later when I realized that none of the makeup stateside looked like *us*. But you would never have known it, because for as long as I can remember sisters have been mixing and matching makeup to get at their desires for what's missing in ways that would really shake up the industry if more of us were "in the house," doing the research and development at mainstream compa- nies. When you think about it, ours has always been a deliberate style, one that is based as much on our verve as a people as it is on our desire to express our

PREVIOUS SPREAD:
Oscar-winning actress
Halle Berry

uniqueness through adornment and change. From the ancient traditions of self-expression through painting, scarring, and tattooing to the contemporary looks of the day, some form of crafting or making up has always been a natural part of Black style. Records of our earliest existence indicate that the traditional use of elements such as kohl, charcoal, and the dust of the earth were used to blacken brows, eyelids, and lips and to paint intricate face and body designs, not only to enhance our beauty but also to indicate the distinction of one's station in life. And mind you, both women *and* men engaged in this fabulosity!

Now, in a future my mother would find amazing, we are having more fun with this inspired touch of creativity called makeup than any other group of women on earth! When I look at sisters such as Mary J., Missy Elliot, Janet, Halle, and others whose attitudes and distinctive approaches to makeup encourage us all to play, I'm more than psyched. If ever there was a time for us to indulge our desires to the fullest, this is it! What is makeup if not another way to communicate style? It's not a need, nor is it a commitment—soap and water will easily take care of anything you don't like about it—and we're all clear that we're fine whether we ever wear it or not, because makeup has nothing to do with who you are, just how you want to express yourself. And you know in the end that's what it's all about: keeping and enjoying the tradition of self-expression.

Understatements

Beauty is a celebration of self, one that first begins on the inside, then manifests itself in the physical. When I sit down at my vanity—a wonderful gift from my husband that brings a sense of ceremony to my ritual of making up—I find serenity and appreciation in carving out this little time at the start of my day to tend what God has given me, so I look forward to it. Ditto for having some of the savviest fabulizers the beauty industry has to offer ready and waiting for me to create just what's in my heart by way of a look. To me how we use makeup is another way of having our say about ourselves. This is why I encourage you to know what you want to express before you ever step up to a cosmetic counter. I see far too many women working hard at making up someone else's face instead of possessing their own. I want you to make up with yourself in mind. When you shop, I'd rather see you approach the experience from the perspective of "This is what I so love about *my* face!" I think this is probably why buying and wearing makeup can become so frustrating at times, because in many instances the person at the counter will suggest a look to you that has absolutely nothing to do with how you feel about yourself or where you want to be when it comes to wearing makeup. So think of makeup as a form of expression that begins in your heart and culminates at your fingertips. The more it begins and ends with you in mind and what you desire, the less chance there'll be for disappointment. Even when celebrities sit to have their makeup done, the process usually begins with the artist asking them, "So what are you feeling today?" Because it's about them and applying the makeup in a way that affirms what the celebrity wants to convey. This isn't to suggest that there aren't tricks and tips from the professionals that you can use—it's not about reinventing the wheel—but it *is* about sitting in the driver's seat and enjoying the ride! So why not go for it? And by all means have some fun.

Star Essentials

Back in the day celebrity makeup artists used to travel to shoots and other calls with a makeup case. Today most of them are wheelin' Louis Vuitton's compact carry-on! Whoever said natural makeup takes a lot more than you'd believe knew what they were talking about! More often than not, though, their booty includes everything from skin care to those savvy digital cameras that everyone travels with to check how the makeup's going to appear when photographed (which they say is a better a gauge than trusting the naked eye), as well as more choices in shades, textures, and tools than you can imagine.

  Then there are those prime essentials that the pros themselves wouldn't be without to make our stars shine—the goods that provide a bit of edge, as well as the staples that ensure a lasting, flawless finish. These essentials include wispy false eyelashes with a base so sheer that they can be worn sans liner, blemish control solutions and drying lotions that can be worn under foundation for those days when skin *isn't* calm, white and off-white eye pencils to make the whites of the eyes appear brighter, brow bleach, highlighting lotions and creams to help the stars get their glow on, and super-coverage makeup formulas for concealing birthmarks and dark spots. Aside from these key items, it's about individual preferences and attitudes about what's essential to giving good face.

  For actress Halle Berry, expressing a look is based on a philosophy of less is more. "I never wanted to take my makeup off and have somebody say, '*That's who you really are?*'" says the busy actress, who sticks to a natural-glam approach even for appearances of the red carpet nature. For occasions like these and photo sessions she enlists the expertise of longtime makeup artist Laura Mohberg, who uses an airbrush to achieve the flawless second-skin finish we're accustomed to seeing her serve. With airbrushing, Berry says, "you don't see the foundation. It's enough to cover any little blemishes, but it doesn't clog your pores or cover who you really are." Her makeup artist also incorporates such tricks as keeping the star's brows "one or two shades lighter so you're not drawn to them and so that they always appear softer." And Mohberg adds that if she knows there's a possibility Halle's going to cry, she uses a water-resistant foundation—"and yes, she had it on the night of the Oscars, so the tears will roll down the cheeks and not take anything with them!" (Brides-to-be, I hope you're listening!) Other essentials Mohberg and Berry favor include the use of sheer iridescent powder on the cheekbones to reflect light, a wash of color on the eyes in a bronze or great nudes, and a cocoa-brown lip pencil and creamy flesh-toned lip color to create a nude stain on her lips.

"Makeup should look like *you*, only better" is the revealing philosophy from a sister who has experimented with more makeup than most of us ever will and who went on to make this possibility true for women of color everywhere, Iman. According to makeup artist Jay Manuel, the supermodel and cosmetic entrepreneur spends most of her days sans makeup in a moisturizer and lip balm. However, Iman believes a proper foundation that's an exact match to your skin tone, with matching powder, are an investment worth making. "For evening appearances and photo sessions," says Manuel, who works Iman's beauty for these close-ups, "it's all about her eyes." This calls for a dramatic smoky look with lots of liner, which her deep-set, perfectly almond-shaped eyes can take without looking over the top. Other essentials include a shimmery powder for the forehead and cheeks and glossy nudes for her lips.

For singer Natalie Cole, who Manuel says loves putting the emphasis on her hazel-green eyes, the star essential is mascara. "Cole has pretty, even skin and can go without foundation," Manuel notes, but she absolutely loves bronzer, which he applies to her cheeks instead of blush and to cast a warm glow on her face here and there. And since the singer has a "really terrific lip line," he forgoes liner altogether, using just a slight stain to put the emphasis on that magical smile.

When asked what goes into making up singer and actress Beyoncé Knowles, makeup artist Reggie Wells says, "Not too much—we just enhance the look of twenty-year-old skin! She knows that it really doesn't take wearing a lot of makeup, that it's about keeping skin fresh." In keeping with this philosophy, Wells says, "I put on moisturizer with a cream foundation, a bit of gloss, mascara, and let her go!"

Tools of the Trade

It doesn't matter how much money you spend or whose formulations you select—without the right tools you'll never get the best possible results from your makeup. A small collection of good-quality, natural-hair brushes that wash well, retain their shape, and won't shed or scratch your skin are essential to the process. Likewise, pick up a couple of durable, dome-shaped sponges (available at department store makeup counters featuring professional makeup lines) for applying foundation and a few latex wedges (at mass market chains) for blending and clean-ups. By all means, toss those compact brushes and tiny sponge applicators that come with your makeup—take my word for it, they just don't cut it! These basic tools will not only aid you tremendously in getting the look you desire, but allow you to apply your makeup quickly and easily, with the most natural results. What's also important to your look is how well you maintain these tools. To prevent dust and bacteria from adhering to them, take the advice of celebrity makeup artist Roxanna Floyd, who styles such famed faces as Queen Latifah and Angela Bassett: "It's best to store your brushes in a case, pouch, or even an inexpensive cylindrical makeup bag, separate and apart from your makeup and sponges to protect delicate hairs and keep them intact." To store sponges and powder puffs—providing the puffs you use are of the washable kind—follow Floyd's mainstay by simply keeping them in a zip-top plastic bag! But, cautions the busy makeup artist, make sure you only store your sponges this way when they're completely dry. "Otherwise it's best to place them in a small box where air can circulate, allowing them to dry naturally," she adds. Finally, make sure to clean brushes and foundation sponges weekly to remove makeup buildup and keep them fresh, soft, and supple. I recommend that you buy latex sponges by the bag—it's more economical—and just discard them before makeup starts to accumulate (within a week). Never use harsh detergents or soap when washing these items; instead, clean them gently with warm water and a baby shampoo or a cleanser developed specifically for this purpose. I usually take a moment on Saturday morning and begin by placing the items in water, applying a small amount of the cleanser in the palm of my hand, and gently swirling them clean, following up with a good rinse. Then I squeeze out the excess water from each item, making sure to reshape the brushes, and lay everything out to air-dry overnight.

Pictured from top to bottom, are several choice brushes that will help you achieve expert makeup every time. Depending on where you want to take your look, feel free to add to them the tools that will get you there and build the collection that will help you express your beauty to the fullest.

Model Lisa Butler

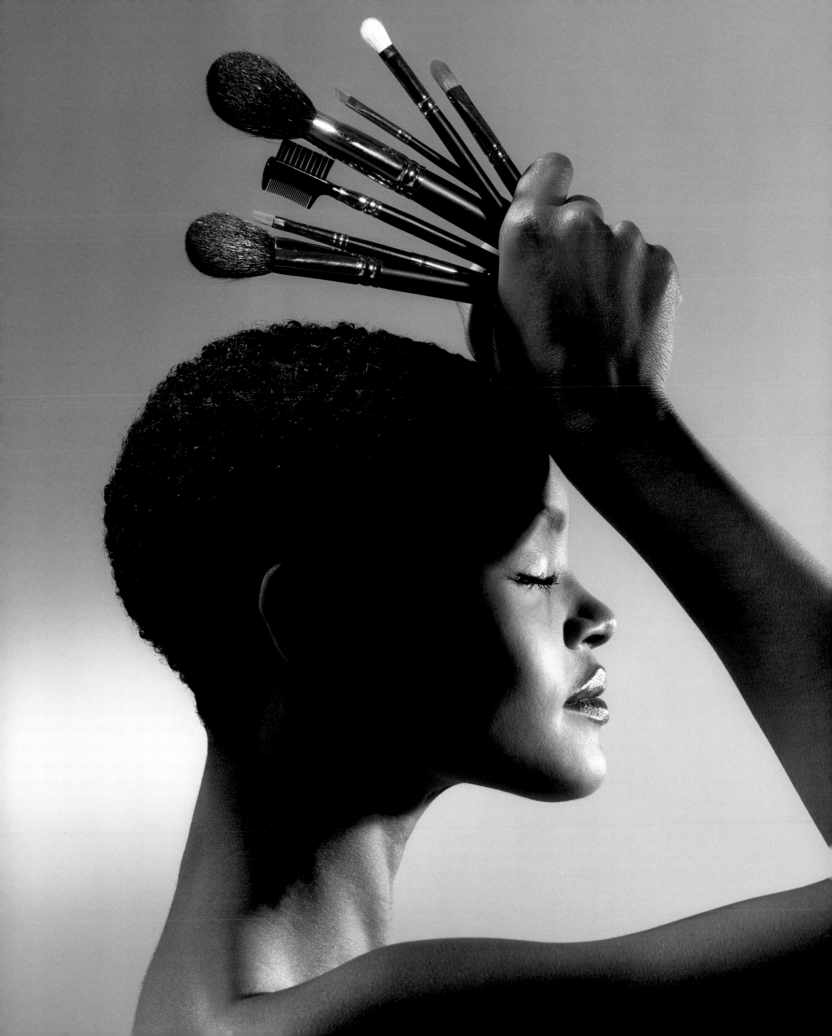

- Flat shadow brush: just the tool for precise application of color to the lids

- Fluffy medium-size shadow brush: great for applying shadow in the crease and unbeatable for applying a sheer wash of color on the lids

- Small angle brush: great for lining eyes or filling in brows

- Powder brush: perfect for face powder or bronzer

- Brow brush/lash comb: excellent for brushing brows into shape and combing and separating lashes

- Lip brush: for a precise application of color and coverage

- Blush brush: perfectly contoured for applying blush accurately

ADDED ATTRACTIONS

The functional items listed below will also aid you in giving great face!

- **Dual-size pencil sharpener: for upkeep of small and large pencils**

- **Tweezers: for cleaning up brows, removing occasional facial hair**

- **Eyelash curler: to get more bang for your buck from mascara by giving lashes a lift upward, thereby making them appear longer**

- **Retractable powder brush: great portable option for on-the-go touch-ups**

- **Blotting papers: to reduce oil and unwanted shine without adding color**

- **Velour powder puff: to apply powder and set foundation in place**

- **Tissues: for blotting lips, cleaning up spills**

- **Cotton swabs: perfect for blending and cleaning up makeup missteps**

Browsing

I've always said brows are "the hood of the face"—in other words, the framework that sets off our facial beauty. It is the brows that punctuate our expressions and play a supporting role in conveying individual style. When all is said and done, brows, not makeup, are the real look makers. Perhaps that's why there are more brow grooming and styling aids available to us than ever before, for without a doubt, a polished look hinges on just how well groomed one's brows are. Beautifully tended brows—those that bear no straggly hairs and are brushed into a neat shape—convey a sense of confidence and order. Brows that are arched and

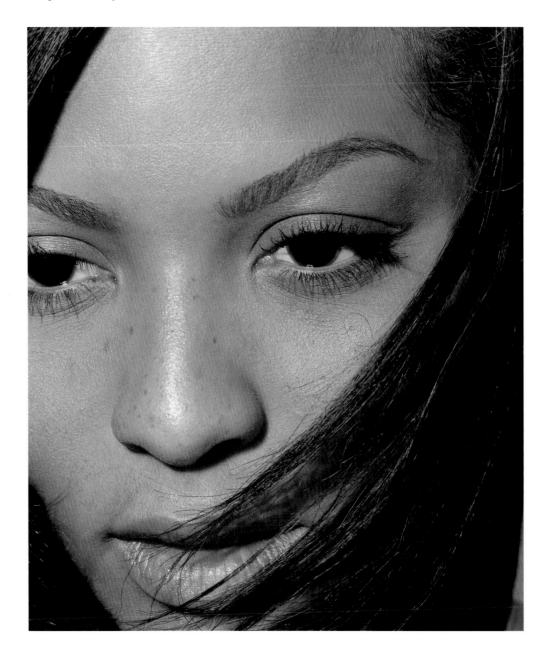

Model
Wendy Brooks

shaped through clipping, tweezing, and/or waxing go a step further and offer a totally new look and even more eye space in which to play with makeup. Brows that are bleached impart yet another dimension, in that they bring a softer glow to the face (and also complement hair that's been lifted to a lighter hue). Even more spellbinding are those sisters who remove their brows entirely, in turn presenting a look quite like sculpture, a bold move I find so soul-stirring!

Quite frankly, I find this area of a woman's beauty so intriguing that I'm always brow watching to see what nuances makeup artists and sisters alike have adapted to tweak their framework. And whether I'm in attendance at the twice-yearly ready-to-wear shows in New York and Paris, on the red carpet at the Oscars or the Essence Awards (where giving good face is always serious business), or on the street, I'm looking to get the close-up on what's newsy. Interestingly enough, what I come back with every time is that brows are about an attitude. On the runway, it's the designer having his or her say-so on the world's top models, but for everyone else, celebrities included, it's another projection of one's sense of self. Take singer Patti LaBelle, whose deep, highly stylized sweeps—always au courant—reflect her confident, entrance-making personality. Or the soulful Lauryn Hill, whose lush, earthy brows speak volumes about her natural, nonconformist approach to life, let alone style. And actress Vanessa Williams's always perfectly plucked and shaded brows, which once graced New York's Times Square thanks to a major cosmetics manufacturer, who perched them on a larger-than-life billboard, denote a penchant for a well-manicured flair. For me, it's always about a slender, tapered brow that's slightly filled in from start to finish. And that's as much about a confident, signature look as it is a need to call together a pair of very sparse brows from years of overplucking! The message here: Don't let this happen to you!

Beyond attitude and desires, serving a look when it comes to your brows also has a lot to do with your lifestyle. According to one expert's theory, we should ask ourselves just how much time we have to devote to maintenance. Some pros maintain this factor should play a major role in the type of shape you're going to present, more so than the technical stuff we often get frustrated by, such as the shape of your eyes or measurement tactics that call for beginning your brows in line with the outer edge of your nostrils, which is fine if you have a Eurocentric nose! "If you're like most sisters and have five or ten minutes to spend on makeup each morning, you don't want to spend it all on your brows, but rather want to groom them just enough to open the eye where the brow bone becomes visible," says celebrity makeup artist Sam Fine, who says this low-maintenance approach calls for tweezing a couple of hairs here and there, or if you have a thicker brow, getting that area waxed. On the other hand, if you have more time to spend, then you may opt for a more deftly shaped brow, something that requires an artful hand, illusionary help by way of a brow pencil or powder, and at first a certain amount of patience. Years of working with the top pros has taught me that no matter where you start, the tools and techniques exist to help you create the brows of your desires.

Shape Up

"Don't be guided by what's in or what's out. In other words, be moved by *what's for you!*" A sage piece of advice from makeup-artist-in-the-know Reggie Wells, who keeps the well-tapered brows of Oprah Winfrey. Truth is, whether you're just beginning to define your brows or need to grow them back in and redefine their shape, it pays to have an idea of what you'd like to express and the maintenance involved, and then enlist the help of a knowledgeable professional. But makeup artist Jay Manuel, who has shaped Tyra Banks's golden arches, urges you to be wary of trusting this aspect of your beauty to just anyone. Says Manuel, "A lot of women will go to the nail salon to have their brows shaped by someone who works strictly on formula." He feels it best to place yourself in the hands of an expert who's going to examine *your* face and bone structure and then make a recommendation. All would agree, however, that if you're defining a look on your own, start small. Begin by purchasing a brow kit complete with stencils and everything you need to assist you in determining your look, or use a white or black eyeliner pencil to draw your desired shape and then remove those hairs that extend beyond the boundaries. If your look calls for hair removal, choose your method carefully. Makeup artists say selecting a suitable form of removal should take into consideration the texture and thickness of your natural brow, as well as your personal preference. "In Oprah's case, we find waxing is better, as tweezing is just torment for her" due to her lush, naturally thicker brows, says Wells. Dermatologist Jeanine B. Downie urges us to take into consideration our skin type as well. "People with dry and sensitive skin have the worst skin for waxing and razoring, which causes bumps for them, and depilatories, which cause inflammation of the hair follicle that irritates the skin," says Downie. Her methods of choice for those of us who fit this profile are tweezing or threading—a method of removal that accurately eliminates hair by the root, using a thread wrapped around the individual hair by the hands of someone skilled at the craft; for those with oily and normal skin types, the best options are waxing, threading, or plucking.

If you tweeze, brow master Sam Fine encourages you to take one hair at a time. "Try not to take two and three. Yes, plucking one hair at a time is a little more painful, but this way you save the hair and escape the holes!" he adds, alluding to what can go wrong when you attempt to speed through the process in an effort to get it over with. I can tell you that over time you do get used to tweezing, and the discomfort diminishes greatly (unless your hair is thick and coarse), but this is one practice where I won't urge you to initially stand the pain by your own hand! However, before you frown on tweezing altogether, what you might try is having it done professionally, or sharing the process with a sister friend. What'll help make it easier is washing your face gently and splashing with warm water so the hair becomes softer, then gliding an ice cube over the area to be tweezed just prior to plucking, to numb the skin. This way you can close your eyes, relax, and allow her to move through the process of tweezing your brows calmly. Once your brows are completed, she'll be able to relax while you reciprocate the favor. Another element that will make tweezing a quick and easy success is having the right tools. Make sure you have a good brow or toothbrush on hand, both to separate and brush brows into shape before you begin and to spot-check the look during the process, as well as a quality pair of sharp tweezers with a flat, angled edge. Using dull, poor-quality tweezers causes brow hairs to break, as opposed to lifting out squarely from the root. Also, make sure to pull the hair in the direction it grows in (something my mother taught me years ago), as pulling it in the opposite direction will cause the hair to break, leaving behind a difficult-to-grasp stub that will only make the process more time-consuming and frustrating. And always tweeze underneath, never on top, as it can really distort your natural line. Manuel, who also favors tweezing, does confess that threading ensures the best shape. If you're about artfully refining your shape, you might take the approach of some sister celebs who go the distance by having their brows trimmed to shorten the length of the hairs and then tweezed and waxed to really sculpt them.

However you choose to edit yours, I ask you to think twice about razoring them into shape, as there is always the possibility of scarring. Furthermore, according to Manuel, with the repeated use of a razor to shape your brows comes an unwelcome darkening of the skin, just as repeated shaving does in any other area of the body, such as the underarms.

Meanwhile, if you decide to keep yours au naturel, make it count by brushing and setting them with a clear gel mascara—better than your typical brow gels, which won't hold curly or coarse hair in place.

Personally, I so love having my brows come together, whether I'm doing the cleanup or I'm in the hands of one of my favorite makeup artists. The beauty of it all is that once you find your line, it's easy to keep in place. However, what I like most at the end of the day when the makeup comes off—even when I rise in the morning—is that groomed brows are the one thing that remain. And that, my sisters, is something to smile about!

Shade Secrets

Whether you choose a pencil or powder to enhance the look and shape of your brows, it's best to go for a great brown for the most natural finish. I also find products made specifically for the brows go on easier and wear better, which is why I advise not using eye shadow or liner pencils to fill in or sculpt your brows unless the product indicates it is suitable for both. What you'll find different about them, particularly the pencils, is they're a bit more matte and moisture-resistant, and they blend easily with your natural brow. A nice plus about the powders, according to Manuel, who favors the use of brow powder as opposed to pencils, is that unlike powder eye shadows, they contain more pigment and no pearl, blend well with your natural brow when applied with a stiff, angled brush, and (unlike some pencils) won't separate from brow hairs and have a detectable presence of their own! Personally, I'm a pencil girl, and I wouldn't be without my little mass market pencil (which matches my dark brown brows perfectly), a good sharpener, great light, and a handheld mirror to set my look. My point is find what works for you and raise a brow! Most of all, keep in mind that you're trying to mimic what's already there, albeit with a little added enhancement, so let that be your guide and choose what helps you achieve that goal easily and believably.

If you wish to lighten the shade of your brows, your salon colorist can perform this service for you with great results. You can also lighten them at home using a bleaching cream specifically for facial hair, available at your local beauty supply store or in the health and beauty aid sections of many of the nation's top drugstores. Lightening brows via a bleaching cream can lift your brows slightly, from a dark to warm brown, or as light as a reddish blond. If you choose to bleach, make sure you follow the instructions, check brows during the process to monitor the color change, and don't be tempted to leave it on for too long, as doing so will cause redness and irritation.

The Goods

Unlike back in the day, when our mothers had only a handful of choices when it came to makeup that worked, cosmetic companies are calling *us* to play with an array of products that meet many of our expectations. We're able to shop our beauty across the board and experiment with color, texture, shimmer, and shine! What a change these entries signal—I remember a time when the last two meant "not for us"! These and other options signal a new day, both in technology and in our attitudes about makeup. Therefore, unlike any other time before, the possibilities are endless when it comes to expressing ourselves through the use of makeup.

Whether you choose to complement your beauty with a full spectrum of cosmetics or simply desire to select the goods that will accentuate certain features, it's important to know what's available to you in order to shop with a keen eye and achieve the results you want. Here, at a glance, is your guide:

PRODUCT	FORMULATION	BENEFIT
Foundation	Liquid	Gives sheer to medium coverage; oil-free formulas are great for oily and combination skin types; water-based formulas are best for normal to dry skin; both give a slightly dewy finish
Compact	Cream	Gives medium to maximum coverage; available in oil-free and moisturizing formulas; imparts a flawless, moist finish
	Cream-to-powder	Formulation gives moderate coverage as a foundation, dries to a matte powder finish; for all skin types
	Stick	Offers medium to maximum coverage; available in oil-free and water-based formulas; gives a semi-matte finish; can also be used as a concealer
Concealer	Solid cream	Provides maximum coverage; great for minimizing undereye circles and dark spots
	Tube	Lightweight cream; gives medium coverage; camouflages minor imperfections, uneven tone
	Stick	Gives somewhat sheer coverage, conceals minor imperfections; sticks can be applied directly onto small areas
	Wand	Gives semi-sheer coverage; best for small areas; is applied onto skin with convenient sponge-tip applicator
Powder	Pressed	Gives medium coverage; sets makeup, zaps shine
	Loose	Gives light coverage and a natural finish; sets and unifies makeup, reduces shine; can also be worn alone
Highlighter	Liquid, cream, or powder	Illuminates skin
Bronzer	Powder or cream	Imparts a warm, sun-kissed color with or without shimmer
Blush	Powder	Imparts a soft, matte film of color
	Cream (pot or stick)	Imparts subtle color with a dewy finish
	Gel	Gives a sheer, translucent glow, with a hint of color

Eye shadow	Powder (pressed)	Opaque color; also doubles as a liner; worn wet or dry
	Powder (loose)	Offers a light wash of see-through color
	Cream	Provides soft color with a natural, dewy finish
Eyeliner	Pencil	Imparts a strong, opaque line
	Liquid	Applied with a brush; gives bold matte or shiny (depending on the formula) definition
	Felt-tip	Great for creating a spidery line; gives the matte definition of a liquid with the application ease of a pencil
	Crayon	Creamier in texture than their slim counterparts; doubles as a liner or shadow
Mascara	Lengthening	Creates the illusion of long, wispy lashes
	Thickening	Gives the appearance of lush lashes
Lip liner	Pencil	Adds depth, definition; prevents lip color from bleeding
Lipstick	Matte	Intense, shine-free, long-wearing color
	Satin	Moist finish, color intensive
	Sheer	Translucent color, delicate shine
Lip gloss	Pot, tube, or wand	Intense shine; see-through or opaque color depending on the formula

Defining a Look

Beyond the right tools and an understanding of makeup formulations and their benefits, all that's required to serve a look is a heart full of expression and a little time. For certain, there'll be days when you'll want to take a more finished approach, from foundation to lipstick, and others where you'll desire to play up certain features; then there'll be those times where you'll take a minimalist approach and simply put the basics in place, such as groomed brows and defined lashes and lips. However you choose to play, be sure to embrace the kind of impact that's confident, fresh, and most of all so easy to wear that you have fun in the process.

Here are two treatments on model Nicola Vassel's fresh-faced beauty: For day, it's a modern look, based on warm neutrals and hints of shimmer. To make the transition to evening, where lighting is generally lower and one's face is often cast in a lovely glow, the eyes were intensified, whereas the lips took on a softer focus. Here's how it came together.

Model Nicola Vassel

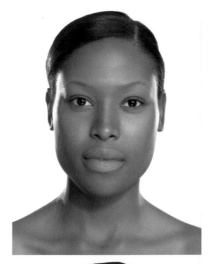

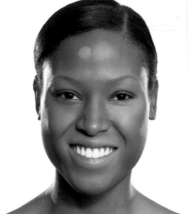

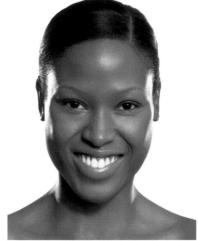

FIRST THINGS FIRST *(left, top)* Skin was prepped using a gentle facial cleanser and an appropriate moisturizer.

PULLING IT TOGETHER *(left, center)* Once the canvas was set, cream concealer, somewhat lighter than her skin tone yet in keeping with her yellow undertones, was applied using a wedge-shaped sponge to hide blemishes and bring up the darker areas of her skin under the eyes and around the mouth.

LAYING THE FOUNDATION *(left, bottom)* A cream base was applied only where needed—to cover the use of concealer, and across the forehead and on the cheeks.

SETTING PRETTY These basics were set with a dusting of loose face powder.

WARM UP *(opposite, top left)* To cancel out the very flat, monotone look that comes about from foundation and powder alone, and to impart a healthy glow, a bronzing powder was used to warm the cheeks and ever so subtly at the temples.

EYE STYLE *(opposite, bottom left)* A single sweep of bronzy shadow, two coats of mascara, and subtly filling in the brows where sparse completes the eyes.

LIP LUXE A muted brown lip liner was faded onto the lips to add depth (*not* color) at the natural line. Lips were then slicked with a neutral shimmer.

ALL SET *(opposite, top right)* Nicola's all smiles about this glowing finish!

NIGHT TRANSITION *(opposite, bottom right)* The easiest way to shift her look from day to night was to intensify her eyes, which were fully rimmed with a matte pencil and layered over with a black shadow for depth and to set the pencil long into the night. Her eyes were given additional focus with a thickening mascara, which makes

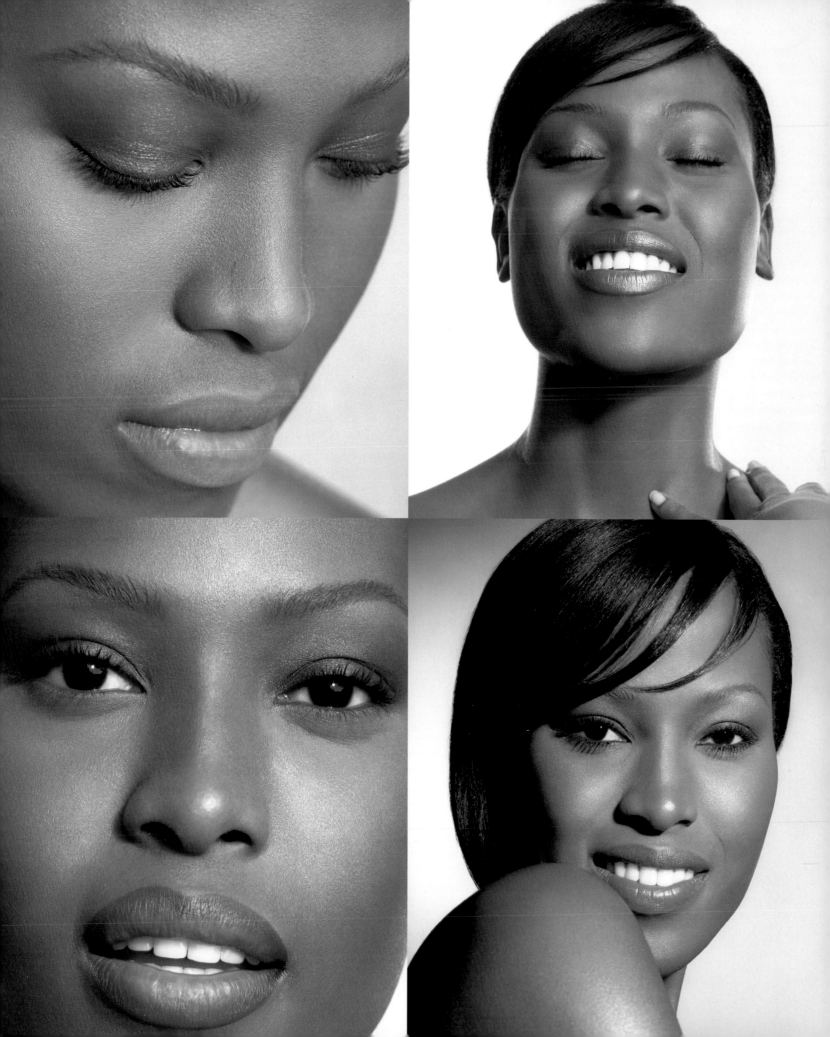

her lashes appear lush and full. With such a dramatic eye emphasis, lips are softened with lip balm, a touch of liner, and a velvety nude lipstick. For you that means beginning by checking your day face to see what needs to be cleaned up or reapplied. A cotton swab is great for smoothing creased eye makeup and clearing away any makeup that's smudged beneath your lower lashes. Zapping excess oil with a blotting paper or gently pressing such areas with a fragrance-free tissue will prime your face for a dusting of powder. Then choose the feature you wish to emphasize, whether eyes or lips, and make it happen. Just be sure to always remove lipstick entirely and smooth lips with a balm before applying color.

New Possibilities!

For me, makeovers aren't about right and wrong—sorry, I just don't believe the Creator sent any of us here wrong! Rather, I think they're about new possibilities. With makeup, it involves taking what you have and shifting it to another level, all the while maintaining a style that's still you. And since we can finally experiment with texture and color, I say why not have a bit of fun? Simply put, the wearing of makeup is another way to express *all* the women you are, perhaps even discover a side you didn't realize existed! When you think about it, in part that's what keeps our eyes peeled to see just how our top celebs are going to turn themselves out at the nation's award ceremonies. We want to know how they're going to express themselves each and every time. And whether it's Mary J., whose style is glam and experimental, Jennifer Lopez, who keeps it romantic albeit with a bit of edge (remember those fur eyelashes she wore at the Academy Awards?), or Yolanda Adams, who's the epitome of classic chic, you know some new dimension is in store. To me that's part of the joy of being a woman, exploring and expressing every facet of yourself for your own distinct pleasure. I remember my girlhood days of playing dress-up and just having the time of my life, without a care in the world about what anyone thought of my getups. And then I grew up and for a moment took that silly pause labeled "What will so-and-so think?" What if I decided to wear purple eye shadow or a blond wig—would I suddenly be the topic of someone's negative conversation or the one they patted on the back because they approved? Well, I've been there and done both, and I'm offering you the same advice I give myself whenever I hit this snag: Who cares? Life is too short to put such simple joys on hold. Frankly, I'm sorry for every moment I wasted wondering what people might think. We should see our beauty in our own mind's eye and confidently explore it to the fullest. And notice I said *we*. This is something we have to claim for ourselves. That in part is the reason makeovers often don't stick. It's not

Model Alina

that they aren't well executed; it's that nothing takes place on the inside, so it's solely about a physical change, which for the most part is fleeting if you can't get your spiritual and emotional arms around it. For example, I did a beauty and fashion makeover for television once, along with *ESSENCE* fashion director Pamela Macklin, on a young single parent. Before the fashion fitting, before the makeup and hair session, we sat down with this sister to quiz her about her inner beauty and empowerment practices. In the dialogue, positive thoughts replaced those that were negative, and then dreams and inspirations unfolded, and so by the time we needed to get down to the mechanics of the makeover process, she was affirmed, fabulous, and more than ready to showcase herself to the world! She ended up getting a wonderful cut, great highlights, defined makeup, and wardrobe selections that perfectly suited her newfound sassy side. So you see, you have to first understand *yourself* before you allow someone else to make an interpretation, and clearly that's an inside job. Here's to giving evidence!

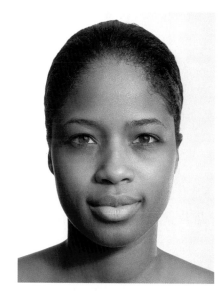

For this ultra-sophisticated take on model Alina, her eyes were cast in the spotlight, with contrasting shadows and a seamless nude lip. Another completely different treatment might have involved putting the focus on her lips using a deep matte stain and a very clean, softly executed eye, using neutral shadows, a bit of brown eyeliner for depth, and a sweep of mascara. Here's how this look came together:

- Brows were bleached to soften their focus and prevent them from competing with

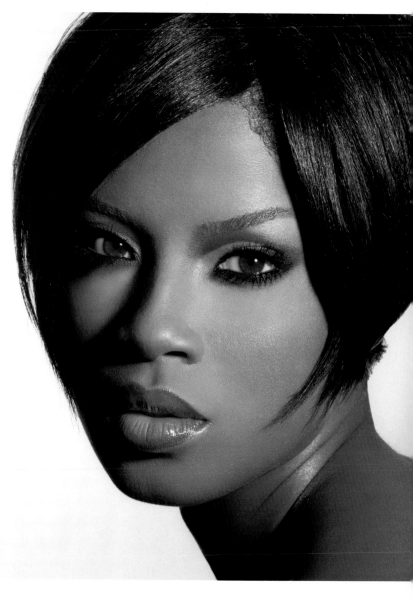

the depth of shadow being used. This also gave the illusion of opening up both her eye space and her face.

■ To prime her canvas, concealer was used under the eyes and around the mouth to balance her skin tone. Then stick foundation was applied and sealed with an illuminating loose face powder for a bit of radiance. To add tone and dimension, powder blush was stroked onto the apples of her cheeks with a large blush brush to ensure that it appeared diffuse.

■ A pale matte shadow was then applied from lid to crease. To create the smoky effect, black and brown shadows were used in the crease and beneath the lower lashes, extending to the outer corners to elongate the appearance of the eye. Eyes were completed with a coat of mascara on the top lashes *only*.

■ Brows were brushed into shape and the ends were filled in and subtly tapered with a brown brow pencil.

■ Lips were defined with a medium brown pencil and a pinked gloss.

■ As a final step, a razor-cut bob was flat-ironed into shape to frame her face.

For model Alwantha Lawson, it was all about achieving a look that says polished beauty, which was accomplished using bronzer and a precise array of shiny deep colors on the lips and eyes. On the other hand, she could have easily taken a semi-matte look, with a neutral eye—shaded from lid to brow—and a matte berry lip. Here's how this look was realized:

Model Alwantha Lawson

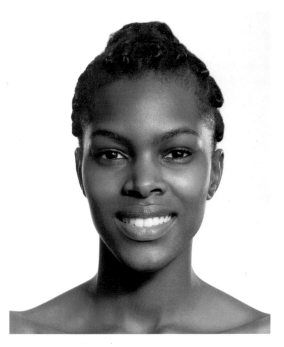

■ To prime her canvas, a touch of concealer was used under the eyes to cancel out natural shadows, followed by cream foundation, which was applied with a damp sponge for minimal coverage. A light dusting of loose powder was used to set the basics.

■ An illuminating bronzer was applied on the eyes from lid to brow bone, as well as on the top of the cheekbone. A cream blush in a dark red hue was used on the apple of the cheeks for dimension.

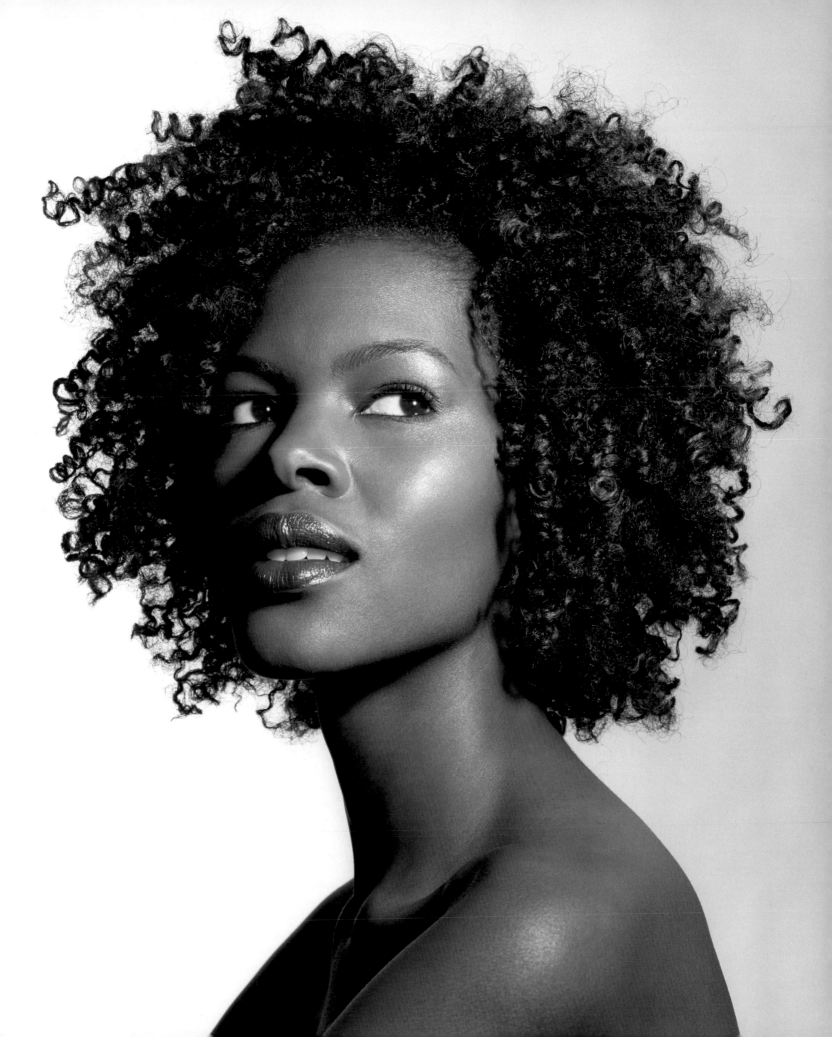

- Eyes were rimmed under the lower lids using a black pencil and completed with a coat of mascara.

- Brows were brushed upward using a clear gel mascara to set them in place.

- A blackened-brown lip pencil was faded in to define the model's natural line and then covered entirely with a burnished brown lipstick.

- Two-strand twists with gilded highlights were finger-shaped to frame her face.

Extra! Extra! Your Look-Great Guide

When it comes to makeup, here's what's key to putting your best face forward:

Choosing the right skin care formulas to prep your canvas

The secret to giving good face starts at the top with these three care basics: cleanse, moisturize, and protect. For makeup to look flawless and wear well, you need to know your skin type, understand your skin's behavior, and treat it accordingly with the proper skin care products. Start your prep with a suitable cleanser, and follow with a moisturizer (a must for everyone) that addresses your complexion and its needs (i.e., check oil, treat breakouts) to help seal in moisture and act as a barrier between your skin and the elements. Make sure it contains sunscreen to protect your skin, even from incidental exposure, and help maintain an even tone. Be sure to apply your moisturizer immediately after you cleanse, and wait a few minutes before you begin to do your makeup to allow your skin to absorb it. By using a moisturizer, you create the perfect base for makeup to go on easily and remain intact. And do include the use of an eye cream or eye gel to hydrate the skin around your eyes, as experts say the skin in this area is fragile and thinner and has fewer oil glands than skin on the rest of the face. I find using a product made specifically for this area is lighter in texture than regular moisturizers and doesn't cause concealer or foundation to separate.

Selecting the proper textures and shades

Expressing your beauty with makeup can range from a look that says nude and lovely to one that's styled to communicate a glam slam. Perfecting either calls for selecting the right textures and shades, because no matter what, you always want to embrace a look that enhances your beauty, as opposed to one that's so overdone it shouts "makeup." For example, I think there's seldom a time when we don't want a look that's healthy and sensuous—glowing here and there with soft hints of color that fall in our comfort zones. Getting there involves selecting the right products every step of the way that in the end result in a finish that's *you*, only better.

Begin by choosing the proper *concealer*, as we all have a little something to hide. To this day, concealers are still a difficult shop for us due to the lack of suitable shades, which is why most experts tend to use a cream foundation to cover and conceal, unless of course for dark circles, for which the opacity of concealers is a must. Experts vary in their opinions on shade selection—some say go one shade lighter than your foundation, some two or three. I always feel makeup artists want to *conceal*, whereas women want to *hide*, something dramatically different, so I go one shade lighter, if that!

From there, it's about selecting a *foundation* that matches both your skin tone as well as your undertone (the underlying color beneath your skin's surface—yellow, red, or blue) and delivers what you want, whether to perfect uneven pigmentation, add a bit of radiance, or help correct skin concerns. For example, some cosmetic companies offer blemish-fighting ingredients such as salicylic acid right in their foundation formulas; others address the concerns of oily skin types with additives such as silicone, talc, and clay. To determine the coverage you'd like, consult "The Goods"—and keep in mind that you might want to switch up your options there. I always say that the face you wear in the boardroom isn't the face you wear on the weekend or out to dinner. Part of the translation comes by way of choosing the right textures, so whenever you can find your shade in different formulations in this category, make that move! To find the right color, select those shades closest to your complexion and apply them along your jawline, then allow a minute for them to dry. Follow by checking them out in daylight, and choose the one that seemingly disappears. And don't be shy about perfecting a second-skin base that's really a fit by creating your own. Simply mix a drop or two of liquid foundation with your facial moisturizer or, for a bit of radiance, mix a drop of a bronzy highlighter with your foundation and apply as usual with a sponge.

Powders should also fall into the scheme of things natural and flawless, so be sure to choose the right shade—one that's not ashy or too red. More often than not, you'll find that a yellow-based powder will fit the bill. Please don't believe the hype about translucent powders—unless you're very fair, those that look ivory in the pan will leave you with an ivory film that has nothing to do with your rich hue! To set your makeup, reach for powders that are gossamer and loose. For T-zone touch-ups, try an oil-blotting or oil-free pressed powder (make sure to blot oil with a facial tissue first) or blotting papers (my favorite); this removes unwanted shine while ensuring that your makeup won't become heavy from repeated applications.

When it comes to *blush*, continue the harmony of a naked, skinlike finish by selecting shades and textures that impart a warm glow. Oftentimes you'll find bronzing creams, powders, or sticks the perfect echo. If you're fair, keep your choices soft, simple, and oh-so-sheer by selecting nudes (with a hint of pink or apricot if these colors exist in your natural tone) to achieve what makeup artists refer to as a "healthy appeal." If you fall into the medium range, keep your choices deliberately warm and feel free to mix in or sweep over a hint of bronze or gold to add a bit of radiance. If you're of a deeper hue, stay in neutral territory—just up the intensity by reaching for brick-oven browns and rich chocolates, or, if your natural undertones are cool, look to those deeps that are woodsy in hue with a hint of color. *Bronzers* also work well on other areas of the face, such as at the temples and chin or overall to warm the skin and give it a rich, healthy glow.

Thanks to today's technology, most *eye shadows* aren't ashy or densely pigmented like those of yesteryear, so I say go on and play! If you're an eye girl like me, you'll love the selection of nudes (ranging from bisque to espresso), especially those with a subtle hint of shimmer; they're available in loose and pressed powders, creams, or liquids to set off a look without seeming as if you tried too hard. Believe it or not, today's see-through formulas will also allow you to enjoy unexpected color and formerly unthinkable metallics—from silver to bronze and a host of shades in between—to further accentuate your eyes.

The possibilities are also great when it comes to *liners*, which are available in creamy, long-wearing pencils or matte powders and a range of shades to further define your eyes. For sure, most of us look to shades of black, brown, or charcoal gray to create the perfect line; however, the idea of layering two colors (such as black over a shimmery gray) to achieve an iridescent effect or placing a powder shadow over a pencil to give depth and set it from dusk to dawn are also great options.

Mascara, in a rich black that looks great on most of us, is indispensable. When selecting a formula, choose one that's closely based on your desires, whether to lengthen or thicken the appearance of your lashes, and your needs, such as a formula that's safe for contact lens wearers, waterproof for when the need arises, or smudgeproof if you find that yours has a tendency to settle in the fine lines beneath your eyes.

Finally, when it comes to your *lips*, you can go from a sheer glossy neutral to the matte red of your dreams without skipping a beat! You can also have fun by mixing textures, even using a loose powder shadow over lip balm and topping it off with a sheer gloss for a look that's so sexy. More often than not, the shades and textures you see on the pages of most magazines are a blend of two products. One thing's for certain, though—*lip liners* should always fall in the subtle category, since their purpose is to define, not frame the lips in an obvious manner. According to makeup artist Sam Fine, shades of brown rule. Here again, it's about selecting a soft texture, as there's nothing worse than a hard, dry pencil that irritates delicate lips and causes you to struggle to get the job done—who needs it?

Seamless application techniques and stay-put maneuvers to keep makeup in place

Today, in this age of instant gratification, the traceless, next-to-natural results we've long desired from makeup formulas are finally here. This alone cuts the process of applying makeup in half! And when you combine these tech-savvy goods with the right techniques, particularly those stay-put practices that keep makeup from fading, separating, smudging, or bleeding, you can't miss! Here's the breakdown.

BASE YOURSELF Remember, foundation items go on more easily over skin that's been moisturized, so never cheat on this important basic. Use concealer on areas where needed (apply with your ring finger, a brush, or a sponge) and blend with a latex wedge. The eye area moves every time you smile or speak, so when you apply concealer there, always make sure to set it with powder, so it won't crack or seep into tiny lines—I've noticed that many makeup artists will do so using a pressed powder and a velour puff. As for foundation, know that less is more, so dot base on the face sparingly and always use a sponge to ensure a flawless finish. For a more natural, sheer finish use a damp sponge. To seal the deal, dip a large fluffy brush into loose powder, tap off the excess, and lightly dust across your face. To add radiance and dimension, as well as avoid a masklike finish that's so uncharacteristic of our skin, you can consider using a highlighter, available in liquid, cream, or powder formulations. If you prefer a liquid, add a drop to your foundation and apply to areas where you want to glow—temples, cheeks, under the brow. Mix cream highlighter in the palm of your hand with your cream foundation and apply with a sponge. Highlighting powders can be dusted on with a large powder brush over your face powder or worn alone.

CHEEK IT OUT It's all about creating warmth using shades that blend easily with your complexion while breaking up the flat, unnatural finish base and powder alone can create. The best way to do so is to subtly apply color from the apple of the cheek and fade it out toward the ear. Choose your preference, whether a cream blush (in pot or stick form), best applied with a sponge; powder, applied with a large blush brush; or a gel stick, the swiftest and easiest to work with, as it can be applied by gliding the tube right over the skin and then tweaking the finish with a sponge. Remember, the goal is to *warm*, not color, so take it easy on the amount of product you use and never, ever try those small applicator brushes that accompany the product—they deposit too much color and the bristles are far too stiff!

SCORE SENSUOUS EYES If it's not your game, skip the rule that says you must look to a tricolor palette. You can sweep on one shade and make your mark or simply place your liner close to the root of the lashes and call it a day. Just be sure to always powder your lids to create a matte surface before you begin, or try a shadow base (developed to keep shadow from creasing). And always use the proper tools so you don't have to work so hard on blending. For powder shadows, apply using the right brush based on the area where you're placing the shadow as well as to achieve your desired finish, keeping in mind that smaller brushes give a more concentrated appearance, whereas medium to larger brushes give shadow a more diffused look. For a smoky effect—the most sensuous look of all—start with a neutral shadow from brow to lid, then place a deeper shade (preferably a medium or deep brown, charcoal gray, or black, depending on whether you want it subtle or dramatic) right under the bone in the crease and subtly extend it out just past your lash line. Follow by applying liner on the top lid—preferably a water-resistant pencil or liquid formula, as they really stay put. Another trick on the smoky end of things is to rim the eyes along the top and bottom lash line with a deep shadow, using a thin, flat brush to place the shadow as a solo look or combining it with the technique just described. When using a cream shadow, dust lids with powder first, then apply sparingly, using your middle finger to blend it thoroughly, and then dust again with powder to set. Complete any look with well-groomed brows.

CREATE LUSH LASHES However you choose to play it, mascara is the one item you want to reach for whether or not you wear any other type of eye makeup, as it's a great form of definition that enhances what's already there. Whenever time permits, curl your lashes first—it's the *only* eye-opener! From there, apply mascara from the base of your upper and lower lashes to the ends, allow to dry a few seconds, then reapply. For lower lashes, I like to use the tip of the wand to gently stroke on mascara and then brush it through. Sometimes I go for a little drama by incorporating a trick I learned from the late Christopher Maldonado, who was responsible for singer Aaliyah's naturally glamorous makeup. Christopher, who also created some of the most beautiful looks for the fashion and beauty pages of *ESSENCE*, came to do my makeup for the Academy Awards one year and taught

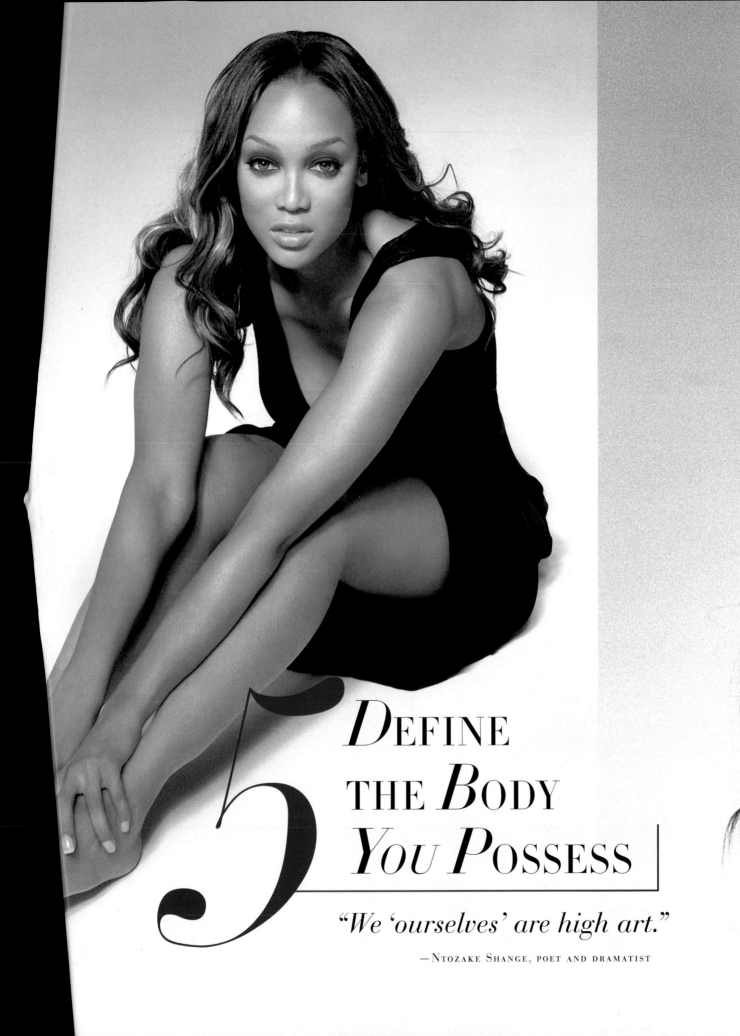

5 Define the Body You Possess

"We 'ourselves' are high art."

—Ntozake Shange, poet and dramatist

me how to make the most of my lower lashes by taking a tweezer to squeeze little groupings of them together while the mascara is still damp to create the most eye-defining clusters. To this day, I just love the impact of this small move!

PAINT THE PERFECT LIPS Rule number one—keep them smooth by exfoliating as needed with a washcloth and a gentle facial cleanser. Use a lip balm that contains hydrating emollients as well as sunscreen, as lips do burn! To define lips and keep lipstick in place, stretch lips into an exaggerated smile and use a lip pencil to trace their natural line. Then powder near the edge of the line, using a small sponge, and apply your lip color with a brush. Another stay-put trick from Sam Fine involves using your lip pencil as a base to both line and fill in lips, then dust with loose powder and apply lipstick. You can also look to transfer-resistant, long-wearing, or matte lipsticks as formulas that go the distance. To keep gloss from bleeding, use sparingly over lipstick and liner. If lips are uneven in tone, dab foundation on before lining and filling in.

SAVE TIME

When the clock is ticking, having the right tools and a palette of sheer neutrals will give you a modern look in five minutes or less, especially if you use a multipurpose product that's meant for eyes, lips, and cheeks. These usually have a bit of shimmer, impart a sensuous gleam, and are practically mistakeproof due to their translucent, often creamy textures. Finish with a hit of mascara to coat your lashes and then set your brows with a clear gel mascara to complete the look.

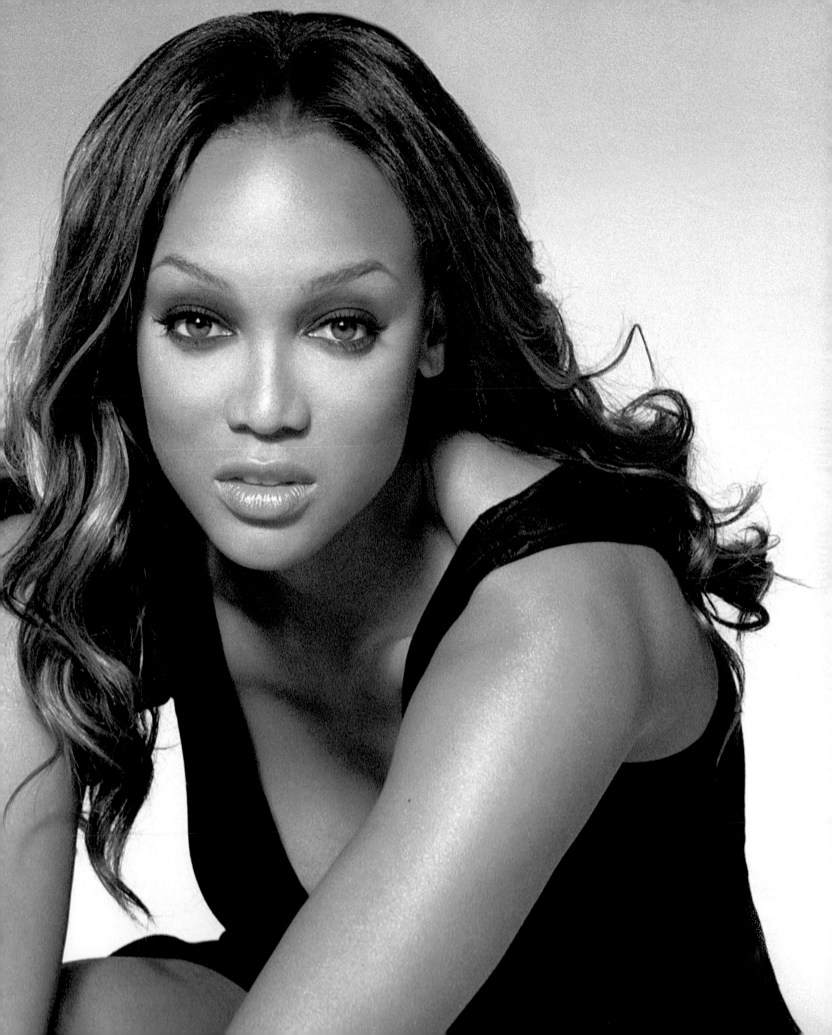

We are living in an age of transformation. Everything, from media messages to products clamoring for our attention within the aisles of the local health food store, is suggesting shortcuts to the beautiful body of our dreams—all we have to do is just try this pill, go on that diet, have this suctioned or lifted or injected or tucked . . . the list goes on and on. As someone who gets the next-next-next word on how to look good and be fabulous from across the nation, however, I'm not convinced that any *one* thing is the be-all and end-all. First of all, I'm a firm believer that a beautiful body is something you have already been given and that maintaining it is an inner and outer pursuit, one that you've got to devote time, energy, and knowledge to, not just throw money at, at least not if you want to play for keeps. Second, you have to intimately know your body before you try to make it conform to something else entirely. And finally, if you want to score real change, you can't even begin to size up where you want to be without first looking at your family's makeup to know just how or *if* you can go there.

Personally, I also think if we seek to understand ourselves the way our ancestors did, this wisdom will guide our beauty and enable us to reap the benefits of good health that outside sources so loftily claim to offer us. This knowledge would also put us in the seat of power and allow us to do the dictating, as opposed to being the ones being dictated to. I know many of us are tired of holding our breath every time we step into a doctor's office for anything from a checkup to a concern. (And more and more of us have dis-ease with somebody's name on it, yet instead of telling the other person the truth or loving ourselves

PREVIOUS SPREAD:
Model and actress
Tyra Banks

enough to move on, we've got a medical prescription, because according to the experts, emotional strain has to manifest itself somehow.) When I look around, type 2 diabetes, obesity, fibroids, high cholesterol, and other health conditions seem to have come home to roost among us, unlike any other group of women in the country. And for many of us, our glorious bodies as sculpted by our Creator, from the full, round, and luscious to the lean and statuesque, are being redefined by the all-too-available ills of fast-food dining. Call it the stress of success or a path at odds with who we are, either way it's time to change the equation and choose that which is in our *best* interest.

"It's about empowering *you* for yourself," says Pamela J. Peters, a specialist in alternative health therapies. It is this belief that continually leads me to look into ancient health practices, such as naturopathy, Ayurveda, iridology, and the like, because I'm searching for a deeper truth and looking to have a body of evidence that's based on sound principles and no compromises. According to Dr. Andrea Sullivan, Ph.D., N.D., a naturopathic practitioner in Washington, D.C., African slaves were the very first naturopaths or healers in America. "We understood that the plants we used in Africa because of the same topography, particularly in West Africa, as we had here in Maryland, Virginia, and Washington, these families of plants could be used for the same things we used them for in Africa," says Sullivan. Naturopathy, which Sullivan cites as part of our birthright and blood right, looks to the cause of a concern, recognizing that we are a total person, body, mind, and spirit. It holds that the total person must be healed in order for us to be well, and it uses remedies from Mother Nature to get you there. Moreover, when it comes to naturopathy, you have to be involved in your own wellness, which is why it fascinates me so. Then there's Ayurveda, a healing science from India that's over five thousand years old, that helps you determine your constitutional makeup and teaches you how to strike a balance in your inner and outer beauty. Ayurvedic physicians are trained in the subtle art of pulse diagnosis, one of their most effective means of assessment, and believe that by gradually changing diet, lifestyle, and the way we process experiences, we actually change from within. Through the help of Pratima Raichur, an Ayurvedic doctor who's also trained in naturopathy, I've come to learn a lot about myself, including which foods to give up to banish the aggravating sinus and migraine headaches I'm prone to, how to achieve my best body through herbs and nutrition, and how to work *with*, not *against*, my constitutional makeup and have more energy. So I more than look forward to my analysis sessions at Raichur's Tej Skin Care Clinic in New York City for periodic updates on the changes without and within and to making those all-important adjustments in my journey. Through iridology, another empowering health path, I'm learning an even greater respect for the intricacies of my body and how it copes with all the stress my lifestyle puts upon it (some of which I'm not even aware of). When I first met iridologist Sally Kravich, it didn't take her long to ascertain that my body was operating "on emergency." I had just returned from several weeks of back-to-back business trips, crossing time zones, eating as best I could on the go, and operating on limited amounts of sleep and high amounts of stress. Her diagnosis included some temporary modifications to my vitamin supplements and my food intake in order to create an internal environment that would allow me to sleep during the night as well as improve the condition of my digestive tract. To further improve my internal picture, Kravich changed my juicing habits to increase my vegetable consumption and negotiated with me to cut out my combination of orange juice and coffee in the morning, which was causing me to be too acidic. When your body is overly acidic, it affects all of your digestive organs, plus your muscular and skeletal systems because it burns up your calcium to neutralize the acid. It also affects your skin's elasticity, and drains your energy. If you think acidity might be a concern for you, your medical doctor can test your levels, but you have to request this specifically. Being acidic also affects your nails, and at the time mine had been peeling like rice paper!

Striking a balance within continues to help me achieve my fitness goals of a strong, tight body that enables me to live the life I desire. The more I learn about my body, the more respect I have for it and the more motivated I become to honor it with practices that increase its strength and endurance. In the last two years, I sent fifteen pounds packing, and believe me, I'm making no provision for their return, because I gained a stronger, healthier body and I'm not willing to fall back into a compromised state of being, dealing with fluctuating weight gain, combating stress through the portals of my refrigerator, and fatigue, all of which stood in the way of being my best self. I've also made this commitment due to my family history of high blood pressure, mild heart attacks, and strokes. Because it's essential to my well-being and overall health, I try to work out at least three times a week, combining both cardiovascular exercise and weight training, along with good old calisthenics. I mix it up with Tae Bo, which takes care of all my frustrations while building great muscle tone, and walking in the city. My eating plan consists of lots of protein, more *living* foods such as vegetables, specific fruits and juices, whole grains, seeds and almonds (as peanuts are fungal and along with other nuts, like cashews and walnuts, stimulate my sinus headaches), and plenty of water. Not that I don't have my challenges. I think rice is the best food in the world. I love it, but it doesn't love me, in that white rice and fried rice both fall into the categories of foods that are gluey and have no nutritional value, life force, or energy. Kravich taught me to have an appreciation for brown rice, which is, as they say, "all good."

The wellness I now possess began as seeds of information placed in my hands, ultimately for me to take and grow. And while reaching your goals in the midst of all that life can serve us may sometimes seem like an insurmountable challenge, the owner's manual to *your* body beautiful belongs ultimately to you. Truth is, we're all facing challenge in some form or fashion, but what it really comes down to is choosing to define the body *you* possess and, as much as it lies in your power, to bring about your desires from within.

Appraising Your Vessel from a Higher Perspective

Few of us go through life without a moment of insecurity about our bodies, or at least some aspect of it. Whenever I hit a moment where I am less than satisfied with mine, I immediately analyze why. More often than not, it has only responded to one or more of my actions that weren't done in the spirit of cooperation and love it thrives on. The Old Testament says we are "wondrously made," and our bodies testify to this truth every day just by the way they perform despite some of the challenges we present them with, whether through a crash diet, unhealthy eating, skipped meals, lack of exercise, or reduced rest. When we're on purpose, however, we understand that our bodies are our temples and they deserve to be tended and well kept. That we're more than a dress size or a shoe size or any other such measurement that doesn't take into account our greatness and importance in the eyes of the Creator, who made us in His image. So let us confirm ourselves in truth. One avenue to higher ground is to set healthful standards, appreciate our uniqueness, and make sure that our inner dialogue and how we regard ourselves are never less than positive.

"Throughout my life, I've bounced back and forth between being comfortable and uncomfortable in my skin," says Tyra Banks. "As a little girl, I was of average weight with a li'l pot belly, and I felt great about myself. As I reached my preteen years, I grew four inches and lost about forty pounds over my three-month summer break—at that point my self-esteem plummeted. Skinny jokes are thought to be politically correct, so I was the target for self-esteem-defeating name-calling," she remembers. Nowadays the model and actress says she's known as a "voluptuous woman," a term she loves being associated with. "I am proud of the fact that I'm twenty pounds heavier than the average model," she adds. Others, like actress Garcelle Beauvais-Nilon, of ABC's *NYPD Blue*, says she keeps her focus on *her* particular body type. "I have breasts, I have hips. When I first started modeling you couldn't have a chest especially for runway, so that was always something that made me think 'oh I'm too big,' and even in adolescence I grew quicker than most of my friends so I'd wear baggy shirts in school to sort of cover up. But I got to the point that this is who I am, and the fact that I have been successful with my body type has made me more confident to work with what I've got. But it is competitive, you have these girls who *are* size two and size zero and we're just not built like that, that's just not us!" Then there's model Keicia Derry, a full-figured beauty who actually started her professional career as an actress at age 13. Derry enjoyed success until age 20, when she became a new mom, after which she struggled with her weight and not being able to get back to her pre-pregnancy figure. Derry says she made up her mind that she wasn't going to put her body through any more of the "sick things I was doing to stay down" or try to compete in an industry where she couldn't be herself. At age 24, the modeling industry welcomed her with open arms. "For the modeling industry I didn't feel I had to be anyone other than who I was," she recalls. More often than not, clients would like her to gain weight, as Derry says she's still too skinny for commercials calling for fuller-figured women! On the other hand, the model says there are still those days when she has to affirm herself when on set with photographers who aren't used to shooting fuller women and can't appreciate their beauty.

Another important facet of judging our vessels from a higher perspective is not to allow outside forces to influence our appreciation of them, no matter how subtle or indirect. In keeping with this thinking, we have to watch what feeds our *spirit*. In a world where beauty is constantly being redefined around standards that aren't based on us, many celeb sisters stay focused and on purpose by standing firm in their truth. "I spend absolutely no time in my day worrying about how other people perceive me in terms of what I look like. I am more concerned with your opinion of my character," says talk-show maven Star Jones. What counts most in her book? "I look good to me and I look good to the people who love me, quite frankly," she concludes. Banks started TZONE—a self-esteem-building adventure for sixty young girls between the ages of 13 and 15 that takes place over the course of one week in the mountains outside of Los Angeles. TZONE allows these girls an opportunity to get away and delve into issues that impact the way they feel about themselves. "Believe it or not, the most emotional discussion that generates the most tears is the night we discuss body image," says Banks. "Even though I put out an image that is very difficult to maintain, I explain to these young women that most of it is smoke and mirrors. The pros spend four hours of hair and makeup time, get the best photographer to light and photograph you and then the best retouching artist to airbrush you to perfection—well, you too can look like a million bucks," she concludes. Banks says she tells them however that at the end of the day, "when I go home and wash my face and remove the hair extensions, I'm just plain old Ty, just a normal girl with tons of insecurities who happens to have a really cool job."

Finally, we have to play a greater role in our health and well-being. Aside from seeing my primary physicians for a complete physical, Pap smear, and mammogram annually, I see a coterie of other experts who help me to manage my temple. Each of them—whether it's my iridologist, naturopathic doctor, nutritionist, or Ayurvedic expert—reveals another aspect of how to take care of my body from within. I'm not alone when it comes to finding the knowledge and practices of Ayurvedic medicine empowering. When I first met actress Halle Berry back in the late 1980s, she had just starting doing a television series, and I was truly impressed (as I continue to be) by her sweet spirit, which looks challenge in the face with a determination to lick it, come what may. Shortly thereafter I had the opportunity to work with her on location and learned that she had diabetes. Working through a busy schedule while trying to maintain her energy, administer insulin, and rest was somewhat difficult, but she was a real trouper and more than mastered the job. But Halle went on to take charge of her health and bring it under her control. The defining moment, Berry says, came when "it got so unmanageable I was living with a lot of fear and wondering when I went to sleep, what if I don't wake up? I decided this is a disease that is manageable and controllable if I just take it seriously, so it was fear and an unwillingness to surrender my life to it" that made her seek to change. Berry says that Western medicine told her, "This is your life and you have to live with it." A holistic doctor told her that didn't have to be so if she was willing to take the risks and try to change it. "So that's what I did. I went on a holistic journey for about three years, saw a nutritionist, and came up with a really good program to wean myself off insulin and onto oral medication. I started to work out and really understand the disease

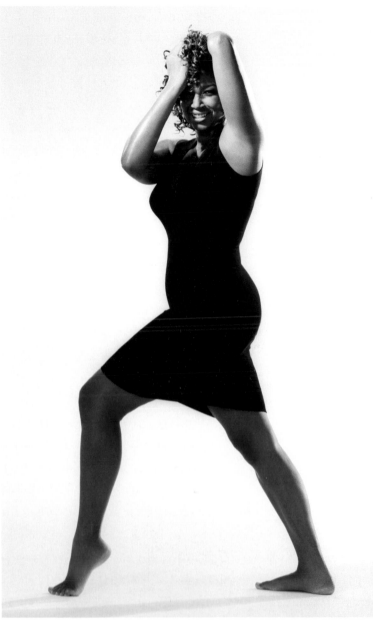

Model Keicia Derry

and my body a lot more," adds Berry. Later she met an Ayurvedic doctor in Hawaii at a seminar, and although that redefined the picture, Berry admits it was quite scary at first. "My Western doctors said, 'If you're going to go this route, then we're going to have to release you as a client because we don't want the responsibility. In our minds this will never work, it's not healthy, it's dangerous, and we don't want to be a part of it,'" she says. Berry remained determined and went on to work with her new doctor, who sent her the necessary herbs, spices, and roots essential to her health every six weeks from India. And she toughed it out. "For about two years it was up and down, high blood sugar days and low blood sugar days and trying to work all at the same time. After about two years he told me it would level out, and sure enough it did."

When I saw singer and actress Vanessa Williams several years ago, she had already been seeing iridologist Sally Kravich for quite some time. Through her exams with Kravich, Williams learned that she needed to avoid processed foods and white flour. "White flour and water when combined make a paste in your intestines, and even if you're eating the right kinds of foods, nothing can be absorbed with this buildup," she says. In fact, Williams went on to say this is true of white sugar and white rice—"all the things that are processed are hard for your body to break down and digest." Williams, who admits that she was much more diligent when she first started seeing Kravich and as a result was thinner and really active, says she learned the value of juicing to cleanse her body, her blood, and her organs, a practice she continues even when she doesn't have the energy to do it at home. "When I'm close to a health food store I'll run in and get it," she laughs. Seeing an iridologist presents another way for you to master good health and well-being. Dr. Maisha Tianuru, founder and president of the Afrikan Center of Well Being, Inc., in Houston, Texas, reminds us that our body temples are the most fascinating creation in the Universe. When it comes appraising them on a higher level, this is the measure. And, she adds, it's important that we recognize that "self-examination must take on our many different bodies; in so doing, we must look at our spiritual bodies, our physical bodies, and our emotional bodies, and then create the time and the energy to support them."

Sculpt: Exercising Your Options

When you get right down to it, feeling good is essential to looking good. How we nurture and push ourselves in the areas of exercise and other physical activities figure greatly. When it comes to shaping and defining the body you possess, it's important to begin by consulting your medical doctor and any other health care professionals that help you manage your temple. From there, you want to again take into consideration your genetic history. Spiritually, you have to be in tune with your vessel and see it for the high art it is. Ask yourself: What will you create from the wonder that you've already been given? Then make choices that are realistic and that you can commit to.

"If I had to pick one thing that does the most toward achieving health, healing, and well-being, it would be exercise," says Therman Evans, president and CEO of Whole Life Associates, a health consulting firm in Elkins Park, Pennsylvania. "If you have a regular exercise program, it's going to elevate your mood, enhance you self-image, make you feel and perform better, and help you to manage your weight even when you're sitting still and doing nothing, because the metabolic rate of muscle is higher than that of fat," Evans adds. Moreover, he and other experts agree that overall, an exercise program actually retards and in some instances reverses the effects of aging. Nevertheless, there was a time when no matter what anyone said to me about the benefits of exercise, I just felt I was too busy to get into it. Instead, I would just waste time and money on the short-lived benefits of fad diets and supplemental foods and beverages. In the process, I watched my body go soft, rebel, and thicken to a capacity that could have had an impact on my heart. Then one day, I expressed to my husband that I would love to bike, if only I had one. Well, sweet man that he is, he bought two—one for the road and, later, a stationary one. I started out riding that summer with my daughter Ashley and loved it. By winter, I was committed. Now I'm smitten, biking fourteen and a half to seventeen miles three times a week, along with other types of cardiovascular exercise and weight training, and I can't live without it! Even on the road, I hit the hotel gym and take to the bike or the treadmill and free weights or any weight-bearing equipment that answers my needs. Aside from the benefits, which highly motivate me, it really makes me feel good to be able to manage this important aspect of my life. I no longer feel I'm too busy to take care of myself in this manner; now it's just a question of balancing my schedule and viewing this form of self-care as a necessity instead of an option. Equally important, because I understand my makeup, in that the women in my family carry excess weight in their abdomen and hips, I've made it a point to discern how to focus my efforts in the areas of exercise and nutrition, as people who naturally put on weight around the middle are known to have a higher risk of heart disease and diabetes, and, equally key, to maintain a keen sense of self-appreciation.

The successful route to a strong, well-defined body, according to fitness pro Kacy Duke, who has helped high-profile celebs like Eve, Foxy Brown, and Iman fine-tune theirs, is to set realistic goals, and equally important, to first show your self some love. "Take a look in the mirror and acknowledge that this is the beginning," Duke encourages, "and accept yourself for what you have and where you are." And instead of beating yourself up about how you look, she reminds us that it's okay to look in the mirror and really get at how you're feeling, even to say, *this is not the body I want right now.* According to Duke, it's important to not accept this acknowledgment as if you're *broken*, but rather to give thanks for empowering clarity, and then look critically at where you want to be. Then give your body the sendoff that it needs by implementing a good foundation that honors you from the inside out. I always say, if you get the mind in shape, the body will follow. Duke says that in order to do so, we must balance three elements of self: emotional, spiritual, and then the physical. "Your approach to getting fit has to be one of truth and we have to watch our words because they are energy, so we have to watch what we say to ourselves," she adds. If you dwell on that which you deem less than positive or only focus on what gets in the way of time to work out, you'll only continue to be dissatisfied and this will impact your ability to be where you really want to be. Instead, set your vision by identifying the desires of your heart; establish specific goals—however small—and what kinds of activities will help you achieve them. At S.W.A.T.T. Fitness, Liggins says she asks women, "What do *you* want?" "It's not what I want, not what the magazines are saying, not what the TV is saying, it's about what you want," she says emphatically, noting that a lot of emphasis is placed on changing women's minds concerning what other people want or what their trainer wants and finding out what they want. "From there," says Liggins, "we build the masterpiece." Once you've determined what you want, then identify any obstacles (read: circumstances you can overcome with planning) or barriers (unpreventable circumstances that impact your schedule and cannot be easily altered), even, truth be told, those excuses that we make, and resolve them with sound strategies. And be grandiose in your appraisal of your vessel with long-term goals that benefit your health and promote total well-being in the process instead of those that are short-term and shallow. For example, it's not about getting in shape for swimsuit season or to be able to wear a certain dress—you deserve better than that. Rather, it's about playing for keeps by accepting this challenge with delight and making a lifestyle change that you can commit to. This is the kind of mental preparation that will take you where you want to be. And be diligent about staying on course by not allowing your determination to be compromised. If you're a working mom like me, you have to schedule this time for self—be it early before getting the kids off to school, or during your lunch hour, or after work. You might even share your goals with a sister-friend, so you can keep each other motivated or share the responsibility of watching the children so you can both get a workout in. You might also share workouts with your spouse or establish a plan that sees you working out with a group of sisters. What also helps is to creatively mix up the types of activities you choose to prevent boredom. When we were children, we used to play and no one ever had to push us to do so, because it was something that we really enjoyed and this consistent form of activity worked out our hearts and lungs, built strong bodies, and contributed to our overall well-being. With the right exercise regimen the same benefits happen, especially if we do that which we enjoy a minimum of three times a week. "Remember, you're making a lifestyle change; fitness is like an adventure. There's many things you can do," says Duke, who urges us to be creative. "You don't have to do what everybody else is doing."

According to the experts, what you want to go for is the perfect blend of cardiovascular, strength, and flexibility training. At S.W.A.T.T. Fitness, the average adventure is 90 minutes, complete with stretching, cardio, strength training, and a full cool-down. "Sometimes we'll be on the sand to jog, sometimes in the mountains to power walk, the women will get their resistance, without equipment, followed by the peace of a cool-down where I have them lie back on their mats, and I meditate with them. I truly believe my camps were designed so women can get their minds *off* their bodies so they can take care of business and do His work!" says Liggins.

When it comes to your health, cardiovascular exercise is the balm! It works your heart and lungs, improves your response to stress, and puts calories through the fire! Whether you choose to walk, jump rope, take up African dancing, bike, kickbox, or skate—or for that matter, engage in any other activity that gets you moving and gets your heart rate up in the process, it's all good, because once you start, your body is going to crave more. The harder you work at it, the better, but if you're a beginner, it's best to start slowly and increase your efforts as you get fitter. "If you're moderately fit and you've been working out, say, jogging, it's time to do more, so maybe you could do a run," says Duke. A sure sign, she says, is if your workout is really too easy. Most of all, know that choosing your most effective form of cardiovascular exercise is a personal one. "If you are a large-size woman, it's best to start off power walking to own your own power where you're in control," says Duke. Once it starts to get easy, perhaps you'll decide to take to the treadmill and do a speed walk. "Most of all, it's important to listen to your body so you'll know when it's time to go to the next level," she concludes.

Studies have shown that strength training (also known as resistance or weight training) isn't just for bodybuilders; it is essential for everyone—but especially women. It protects bones from osteoporosis and prevents the age-related decline in lean body tissue that leaves us weak and many times overweight. No matter what your age or fitness level, weight training will aid you in your goal for a tighter, stronger body. It is also said to improve balance, ultimately reducing the risk of bone-breaking falls. As we age, our muscles shrink and fat takes their place. This leads to a slowdown in our metabolism and weight gain. Weight

DEFINE THE BODY
YOU POSSESS

training can reverse this process, increasing your muscle tone and diminishing your fat stores. It also imbues you with a sense of well-being. The nice thing about it is that you don't have to invest in expensive equipment. I began with my own body weight and a resistance band, then a few hand weights of varied poundages and an exercise tape. What's most important, though, is maintaining the proper form as you exercise and using the right weight for your level of strength. For example, you should feel challenged when using the weight, not overwhelmed. Key to the process is to start slowly and gradually increase your reps and the amount of weight you use and to limit your workouts to two or three times a week with a day off in between to allow your muscles time to recover.

Flexibility training is often neglected because its benefits aren't always immediately apparent. But considering that the average adult loses 40 percent of their flexibility between the ages of 20 and 70, I know it pays to take those few extra moments at the beginning and end of a workout to do those all-important stretches—to me they're like a deep breath for my body, mind, and spirit. Given the way we live, it isn't as much about being able to reach your toes as it is for combating the tension that's almost a constant in parts of our bodies, such as the neck and shoulders or the knees and legs, or the prolonged periods we spend in a single position that promote stiffness or a reduced range of motion in our joints. So whenever you can get in a moment to stretch, whether in the middle of the day, after work in a yoga or stretch class, or at night after a hot bath, do so—it's a small investment with a big payoff.

When all is said and done, the latest research shows that exercise is the real fountain of youth, as it rejuvenates one from head to toe. Moreover, it enables us to live the lives we want and to possess the stamina and strength we need to do so. So think of it as a wise investment for preserving your temple. And be encouraged—says Liggins, "a winner is a winner from the start and only winners start. Losers don't even get there. When you fall off you can always enter the race again. Every time you fall, you learn something, so learn from it and get back in the race." Most of all, remember to "enjoy *your* process," she adds, while you're on the way from where you are to where you want to be, "as once you get there, it's not half as much fun."

Sweet Inspirations

The perfect workout regime that helps one to achieve goals varies from woman to woman and is motivated by different reasons and seasons in one's life. Nevertheless, the essential ingredients are commitment and options that you enjoy that will fulfill your desires for body, mind, and spirit. Here are some inspirations from sisters who've found their path:

Model Karen Alexander: "I always assumed that I was going to live this regimented life and life isn't like that. So I joined a gym that has branches everywhere and whether it's fifteen minutes on the treadmill or time to take a class, it's helped me. I even see the difference in my skin; it's not as sluggish-looking. So this access ends up costing more, but I'm willing to do without a new designer bag to be able to have a gym that I can go to everywhere, at any time."

Model Keicia Derry: "I started working out to be strong. I have a yoga tape I use at home, and I also go to the gym at least three times a week. Exercise for so long was compulsive with me, but after my daughter was born, I made a decision to be healthy so I wouldn't pass any junk onto her. So now my daughter and I walk for hours and we love to swim, so we're exercising, but it's much more than that; it's a time for us to bond."

Actress Halle Berry: "Having the real need to exercise regularly for my diabetes has helped a lot. My personal trainer has put together a routine that consists of a half-hour of cardio (running), fifteen minutes of sit-ups to tone the abdominal area, free weights and Nautilus, and about fifteen minutes of stretching to keep the muscles long and lean and from being too masculine. I also do Pilates and a little yoga for variety. Definition and muscle tone are good, but I never want to look like I just work out in the gym—I don't find that look attractive and feminine to my eye—as a woman I just never wanted to look like that."

Model and actress Tyra Banks: "I was the passenger in a car accident a few years ago and as a result, I've been left with a recurring back injury. My chiropractor suggested Pilates as part of my physical therapy. At first, I dodged signing up because the Pilates apparatus looked like something from a torture chamber. But I finally agreed and now I am hooked! Shoot, I am addicted! I'm getting a six-pack, muscular arms, and strong calves (I've always had chicken legs). I am in love with Pilates!"

Fashion buyer Jennifer Thread McHenry: "Two days a week I lift weights and three days I hike or run on the beach and do the famous Santa Monica stairs. I love exercising outdoors; that's where I gain the most benefits physically and emotionally. I truly feel the endorphins. After about five miles I have forgiven whoever I felt has done anything to me and in the end I want to run to my car and tell them it's okay."

Actress Garcelle Beauvais-Nilon: "For me it's staying spiritual, working out to the best of my ability. I work out two to three times a week if I can—Pilates three times a week and cardio on the treadmill twice a week. As we get older, I see things changing and now I realize I better get on that treadmill! But you just have to stay focused."

Actress Latanya Richardson Jackson: "You have to exercise—there's just no way you're not going to do that—and drink plenty of water, that's the truth. And the older I get, the more I'm clinging to the truth! The boot camp that I'm involved in—I'm addicted to it. And I've realized that for whatever reason and no matter what the level of stress I'm under, my body required this level of work to be happy."

Fabulously Fit Divas Who Rule!

When it comes to looking good and feeling fabulous, there are some sisters who've got the keys in the palm of their hand through exercise. Without hesitation, they'll tell you there are no secrets—you've got to get down to the business of maintaining your body with an informed intent and then get to work! Meet four amazing women who did and be inspired.

KIMBERLYN PARRIS Twenty-two-year-old Canadian Kimberlyn Parris ran track for about eight years. Today, as a professional model in New York City, she's traded in her track suit for edgy workout gear and weekly Tae Bo sessions to keep her body well toned and up for the demands of modeling. Parris, who believes the earlier you start working out the easier it is, also hits the gym once or twice a week for cardio and weight-bearing exercises. She basically likes to stay on the move and says she also enjoys walking all over the city, including to her many castings for possible assignments. What motivates her? "I look at all the things that I've accomplished, making my family happy, and thank God every day that I could do what I could do." *Motivating tip:* "Make it fun. Going to the gym doesn't have to be laborious, where you do the same thing over and over again. Change it up—don't get stuck in the same routine!"

DANIELLE CARRINGTON As a newlywed, 40-year-old Danielle Carrington has the best of both worlds, being married to a wonderful man who also trains and challenges her six days a week in the gym. Most mornings they're there by 5:30 A.M. and weight-train for an hour, working different body parts each day. The busy retail assistant from Los Angeles says she started working out two years ago, feeling that she needed to get healthier—no small challenge for Carrington, who has Graves disease and is asthmatic. "Working out has helped me tremendously, but I have to watch my triggers. There are so many days when I don't feel

STYLE TIP

Getting to the gym can be a feat in and of itself sometimes, especially if you're heading there before or during your workday! Without question, time is of the essence and pulling a look together when you're done calls for a strategy of shortcuts to get you there. Here's the way to go:

- Keep your gym bag packed with ultra-portable staples or those that are multipurpose (a makeup crayon for eyes, lips, and cheeks, a palm-sized tin of shea butter to double as body moisturizer and hair treatment) to help you emerge looking fabulous in no time. Another solution: Stock up on mini-sized items like antiperspirant, shower gel, body lotion, whatever you find essential, when you're in your local health and beauty-aids store. You can also decant your favorites into travel-size containers.

- When you're working out, your hair gets its own impact from perspiration, which is drying and can cause breakage. To combat these damaging effects, it's best to cleanse your hair post-workout with a shampoo that's gentle and safe enough for frequent use. If your hair is relaxed, you can alternate shampooing with rinsing the perspiration from your hair. Be sure, however, to always follow up with a moisturizing conditioner and dry hair on a low setting. Keep your look simple with a coterie of styles that you can achieve in minutes, such as chignons, ponytails, or short cuts that allow you to gel, shape, and go, or look to such low-maintenance dos as braids, twists, and locks.

- Think fresh and simple when it comes to makeup. Aside from keeping your stash minimal and your look easy with a multipurpose crayon or compact, try setting your look with a tinted moisturizer or a foundation stick and blotting papers to zap shine and oil and mascara.

like it and then fifteen minutes after I'm there I'm pumped." And the biggest surprise about exercising? "That I might enjoy it. I hated going, you couldn't get me there if my life depended on it, but now I'm addicted," she says. *Motivating tip:* "[Before I began working out,] I didn't have as much energy and I was always craving more—from coffee and soda. When I first started exercising, I walked everywhere because it felt good and you can see the changes that your body goes through even when you're getting a minimal amount of exercise—so walking is huge! Anyone who might be looking for energy should start out with a mild routine; if they enjoy sightseeing, walking is something they could incorporate into their day."

ERNESTINE SHEPHERD, a Maryland elementary school teacher, started her move toward a fit life at age 55, under circumstances many of us can relate to. "My sister and I were trying on bathing suits one day in a fitting room and took a look at each other, had a good laugh, and decided we needed to do something!" Today,

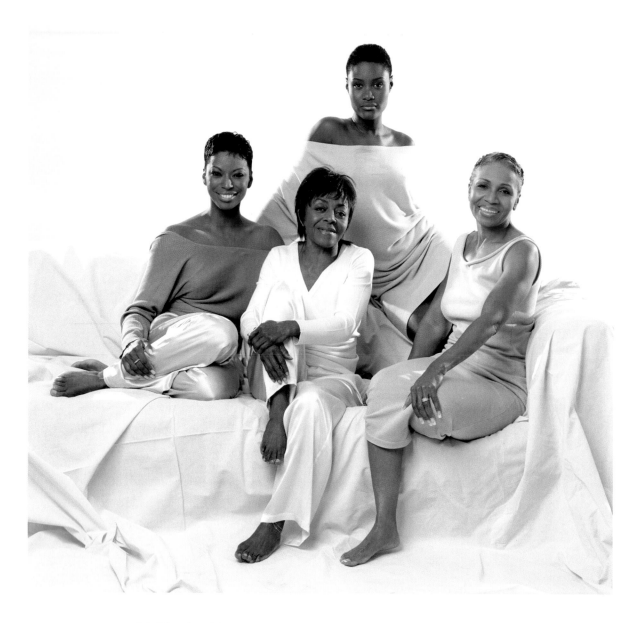

at 66, Shepherd has an exercise routine that begins at 3:00 A.M. *every day* and includes walking ten miles weekday mornings with an additional two hours spent in the gym each afternoon, where a professional trainer helps her with body-building exercises. On weekends she ups the trek an additional ten miles. As for the rewards? "I've noticed the definition, and I feel stronger, younger, and have much more energy," she laughs. Shepherd, who also teaches senior citizens aerobics and weight lifting at a nearby gym twice a week, says she finds it empowering to receive compliments, especially those that lead to "How old are you?" She says women usually want to know her routine, and from there many become her clients! *Motivating tip:* "You don't always have to go to a gym. You can do certain things at home, like take half an hour and, using some small weights, do arm movements, work your shoulders, do squats, and if you do that every day (and eat the proper foods too), you'll see a change."

MORJORIE NEWLIN When 82-year-old bodybuilder Morjorie Newlin decided to weight-train—at age 72—she did so because she found out that weight-bearing exercise could offset the effects of osteoporosis and allow her to be strong enough to do the things she desired to do. "And to be as independent as I wanted to be," she adds. Newlin, a retired nurse, also didn't want her children to take care of her, so she got the go-ahead from her doctor and then set out to look for a gym where she could be trained properly. Was it tough at first? For sure, and there were setbacks. "My appendix ruptured a month after I started and I was hospitalized for about eighteen days, but I went back into the gym three months later!" The Philadelphia native was more than determined to define her body on her own terms, and today, at 102 pounds, she bench-presses along with the "fellas," as she puts it, in a no-frills gym! "I can bench-press sixty-five pounds without a spotter and ninety pounds with a spotter. However, I think I should be able to do more!" When all is said and done, Newlin, who competed in the World Physique Federation competition held in Italy in 2000, winning the Miss Universe Masters, and placed fourth in the masters competition in France in 2001, competing alongside those age 35 and up, says it just makes her feel good to be strong and to be able to do what she has to do. *Motivating tip:* "You've got to work out to keep your muscles and your bones strong, with cardio and just enough resistance. So many women are concerned about getting big and muscular. Women who are doing that are doing so because they want to!"

Motivations for Making Exercise a Priority in Your Life

It's never too late or too early to start exercising and reap the benefits of good health, great energy, vibrant skin, and a tight body that's fit for life. What's key is finding something you like to do and then committing to it. Actress Michael Michelle plays basketball because she enjoys it, while appreciating the fact that it's a fun way to maintain her lean figure. Aside from working out with her personal trainer, Kacy Duke, model Veronica Webb makes a point of doing things that she enjoys as well: "I take ballet, yoga, and jazz dance classes." Moreover, Webb cites exercise as essential to more than a great body. "My mental health is a combination of my religious background, therapy, and *fitness*," she notes. To put you on the move or keep your interest from waning, experts say, it's best to do an assessment in the nude. Then it's time to be specific. Where are you now and where would you like to be? Do you want to improve your overall tone or tighten your abs? Are you ready to enter a marathon or a walkathon? Perhaps it's time for your class reunion? If the latter is where your interest lies, realize that this is a short-term goal, one that won't help you achieve the body you desire for keeps. Besides, you deserve better.

Now it's time to write down your goals and set about making them happen. From time to time I check in with a personal trainer to tailor my moves (an affordable solution) for specific results. You might do the same, or if this is your first time, book an hour and ask the trainer to help you plot a course to reach your desires on your own. Then set yourself up to succeed guided by the following:

- *Vary your workout routine* and be sure to include other like-minded sisters in your activities as often as possible.

- *Be clear about your objectives.* Determine what you're going to do as well as when and how.

- *Tend your goals.* Focus on small accomplishments and particularly on the process, as opposed to checking the mirror for results.

- *Be realistic.* The old adage "Whatever's worth having is worth working for" is still true. Hang in there!

- *Stay positive.* Don't lament the difficulty or the lack of visual progress; instead celebrate your commitment to yourself, and keep pushing!

- *Get your family's support.* To me this is key. If they're not in gear with you, it makes accomplishing your goals that much more difficult. So whether it's a walk in the park or a weekly swim class, make sure they support your efforts—or join you!

- *Be consistent.* If you keep at your choices, results will come.

The Bottom Line

Oftentimes when I'm out talking to marketing executives in the beauty industry about us, the subject of aging comes up along with the question "Just how do Black women age?" The answer to that is "Very well, with minimal wrinkling, a few flesh moles, and a loss of firmness very late in the stages of our lives!" This loss of firmness, however, doesn't just show up on our faces—in fact, it shows up on our backsides and, depending on your lifestyle, sometimes sooner rather than later. Funny thing is, it sort of creeps up on you, because (a) who among us thinks that we have to do anything to tend what is a sweet given? and (b) within our culture, we don't obsess about our bodies—so who's checking to see whether their cheeks are still as high, round, and cut as they used to be? When you get right down to it, our derri-

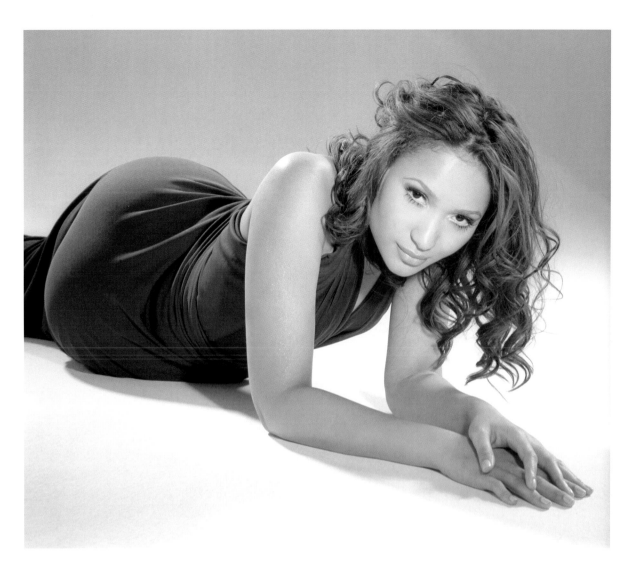

eres represent yet another aspect of our beauty that we're more than proud of. While I spend considerable time working out, I'm not trying to take away my heritage. Rather, I'm toning it with honor because this is who I am and I like what I see.

Keeping a firm backside calls for some specific exercises, though, that you can easily slip into your workout regime. What's basic, according to Valerie Liggins of S.W.A.T.T. Fitness in Los Angeles, is "a minimum amount of cardio (thirty minutes three times a week), squats, lunges, and then constantly varying your routine." It's also important to challenge yourself by increasing your reps. A good rule of thumb is to begin with a set of ten and then gradually work up to twenty-five. Liggins says it's also important to make sure, when you're working through these specific exercises, to stretch and squeeze and really establish a "muscle-mind" connection. So go ahead and strut your stuff! Here are ten tips that'll help you mix it up, prevent boredom, and keep your muscles challenged:

IN THE GYM: Hit the StairMaster, StepMil, or take a Spinning class

Model Immaculee

ON THE GO: Take the stairs two at a time whenever possible

GET DOWN: Leg-raises work the entire rear without fail! To begin, get on your hands and knees, with your back straight and your head lifted. Lift your left knee off the ground and raise it as high as it will go keeping the knee bent and your heel pointed toward the ceiling. Lift it up and down for 10 reps making sure to keep your tummy tucked and your back straight. Lower your leg and repeat on the other side.

AIM HIGH: Take up kickboxing, Tae-Bo, or simply jump rope; all will help lift and define your butt.

PULL UP A MAT: Do prone leg lifts. Lie down on your stomach, with your chin resting on your arms (crossed in front of you) and legs in an extended position. With your hipbones pressed to the mat, lift and lower your right leg as high as you can without releasing your control and arching your back. Do 10 reps, then switch to the other side and repeat.

TRY AN ALTERNATIVE APPROACH: Try Yogilates (a combo of yoga and pilates), or take up ballet; both will give you a firm butt and long, lean muscles overall.

HOLD TIGHT: Squeeze, squeeze, squeeze whenever you think about it to keep muscles in check!

WALK: Hit the park, and try walking lunges or in a confined space do stationary ones. Here's how: Stand with your legs together, abdominals tucked in, feet forward, knees slightly bent and hands on your hips. Keeping your buttocks tight, step forward with your right leg, placing your right foot firmly in front of you. Bend your back knee toward the floor, dipping as low as you can without touching the floor, placing your weight on your toes. Return to starting position by pushing off your right foot, stepping back, and repeat.

PUSH UP: Get on a leg press machine in the proper position and (using the level of weights that you're most comfortable with) lower the weight as far as possible, allowing your knees to come to your chest, making sure to keep your back flat. Squeeze your buttocks as hard as possible and return to starting position.

KICK BACK: with diagonal leg lifts. Pull up a chair with its back to your right side in a standing position. Place your right hand on the chair for support and your left hand on your left hip. Contract your abs and squeeze your buttocks. Then point toes on your left foot and press your left leg back at a diagonal angle, lifting it as far as you can. Lower it and repeat for 10 reps. Switch position and repeat on the other side.

Fueling Your Mind, Feeding Your Body

Diets and food fads come and go, but what I've learned over the years from much trial and error is that there is no magic cure for maintaining health and losing or stabilizing your weight. The solution is tried and true: Set realistic goals and concentrate on healthy food choices. Achieving any physical goal comes by way of a focused mind-set. Once you turn that corner, success is yours. When it comes to managing your nutrition, the healthiest diet is one that includes lots of plant foods, protein, whole grains, water, and healthy fats—not one that puts you in bondage with restrictions that could be hazardous to your health in the long run.

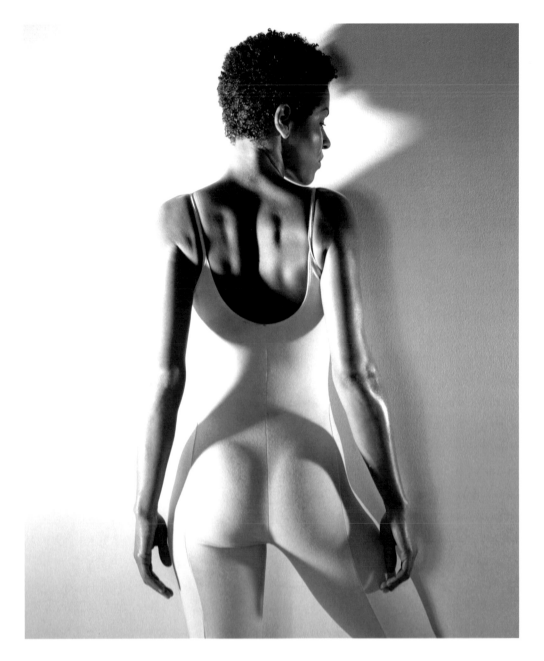

*Model
Rochelle Hunt*

Woman to Woman . . .

My brother and I often have a good laugh about the foods we used to sigh for. Growing up our diet was chock-full of those Southern delights that made you want to run home from school and dig in. From fried pork chops and smothered chicken to sweet potato pies and deep-dish cobblers—our grandmother kept our kitchen humming pretty much from Sunday to Sunday. We often had *company* (as my folks used call our guests) and so Granny always prided herself on having something scrumptious to offer them. Back in the sixties, Newark was truly a mecca for jazz greats and Mommy's industry friends; members of various bands would come by for a visit or even bunk up for the night. But whether it was show biz folks, Mother's swanky girlfriends, or any of the various "play" aunts and uncles who made up our little extended family didn't matter—everyone got the same hospitality, down-home cooking, and lively conversation. Suffice it to say, my siblings and I always ate well and were often treated to additional sweets from our favorite candy store. Looking back, I've come to realize that feeding our taste buds was a big priority and for a long time, that was a habit that was hard for me to break. Moreover, I can clearly see that our minds were quite conditioned to believe that food was a comforting reward, and that more often than not, it was quite a social tool as well. Interestingly enough, no one around us ever made the association between food and the state of one's mental and physical health—perhaps your dress or clothing size—but not your internal well-being. Oh yes, we grew up knowing the importance of eating your vegetables, however, no disrespect to my folks, the way they were prepared—let's just say that the nutrients had come and gone! Back in the day, the connection between food and one's health was usually made by a doctor, albeit a little too late, once he or she began treating you for a medical condition. For as long as I can remember, both of my grandmothers had high blood pressure. Later, my mother and father had this condition as well. Often times I would hear them and others who came to the house say, "the doctor says I can't have this or I have to stay away from that." Other times I would observe my mother on one of her restricive diets aimed at losing five pounds fast and make a totally different connection about food. By the time I came of age, I had my own relationship with it, from the very personal, uninformed thinking of a model trying to stay unreasonably thin to survive in the business, to the equally disempowered one of life in the fast lane as a working girl eating on the go, often stress-related, chock-full of quick, empty-calorie foods followed by short-term periods of dieting when I was trying to pick up the pieces. Thankfully, I didn't pass this kind of behavior on to my children. In fact, I took great pains to see that home-cooked, healthy meals were served across our table and that fast food was picked up only on those unexpected occasions when neither I nor my husband were able to cook. But on a personal level, becoming educated about food to the point where I'm learning to eat unto a purpose, with the goals of optimum health and longevity in mind, as opposed to that which solely serves my palate or any other alternative purpose, didn't happen overnight. And, I'll tell you, given my lifestyle, I still have to stay focused to remain on this path. But again, thanks to my temple management team I'm clear about which foods to eat and those to steer clear of—particularly starches like white rice and white potatoes, as well as dairy products and bread, all of which throw my *doshas* off balance and cause me to gain weight easily. According to nutritional consultant Oz Garcia, we all must avoid consuming what he calls the killer foods. "Starches—the dangerous provocative starches—including foods such as pizza, pasta, and bread, that make you bloated, fat, and irritable: these are foods that alter you metabolically," Garcia says, adding that they should be eaten only once in a while.

I try to avoid sugar at all costs and that means scrutinizing foods with added sweeteners like sucrose, fructose, maple, fruit or corn syrup, dextrose, glucose, maltose, and of course honey. With the exception of molasses, which has some iron and calcium, these additives represent empty calories and zero nutrition. Moreover, consuming too much sugar (more than 18 percent of your caloric intake) compromises the absorption of calcium, iron, and zinc. For women in particular, this is too high a price to pay for an overzealous sweet tooth! Overall, I'm striving to eat more protein such as chicken, turkey, fish, beans, tofu, and egg whites, along with lots of fruits and vegetables—preferably raw or steamed. The payoff here is that fruits and vegetables are low in fat, big on fiber, and full of natural chemicals that can help protect the body against various diseases. Experts urge us to eat five servings of fruits and vegetables a day, and the latest data indicates eating nine or more servings—especially of vegetables and fruits with colorful skins (rich sources of protective phytonutrients, antioxidants, and beta carotene)—for optimal health and antiaging benefits. Getting your daily servings of fruits and vegetables is a lot easier than one might think. It just requires planning ahead and shopping accordingly. Both can be diced or chopped and stored in zip-top bags so they're ready whenever you are. I often freeze my fruits and pop them in the blender with a little protein powder and ice for a breakfast—or any time I need a boost—smoothie. Other times, I'll have fruit with my cereal or at my desk in the evening so I don't arrive home ravenous before dinner can be prepared. Leafy green salads, often twice a day, are also a staple. On the go, a bag of crunchy carrots easily satisfies my need to snack. In addition to eating my vegetables I also juice them. I'm not as diligent as Erykah Badu who juices two to four times a day, but knowing the benefits, I'd sure like to get there!

Badu, who's a vegan, has been juicing for a long time and has a regimen that includes the addition of wheatgrass (a blood purifier) which she proclaims is like Drano for the system! She also makes sure to eat lots of raw salads, sea vegetables, and, to address her anemia, beets, turnips, and blackstrap molasses—a miracle combination she learned from Queen Afua, of The Heal Thyself Living Center in Brooklyn, while she was living in New York. In addition to Afua's remedy, I'm trying to include more chlorophyll-rich greens in my choices, like kale, spinach, collards, and the like, a sound piece of advice given to me by iridologist Sally Kravich, due to my tendency to be anemic. Chlorophyll is the closest composition to blood and so in addition to getting it through juicing I also take it in supplement form. And speaking of supplements, in addition to taking calcium supplements, I've replaced cow's milk, which Sullivan reminded me is for calves, with soy milk.

Making the change to a way of eating that will promote wellness was a question of fueling my mind with the right information and recognizing that this kind of commitment was in my best interest. What kept it going was the transformation that I began to see, both in terms of my energy levels and overall well-being. In the process I also gained a deeper understanding of myself and a new respect for my constitutional makeup and that continues to encourage me to work with it as opposed to against it. And believe me, every time I cheat or go against the grain, I pay for it, with bloating, headaches, lackluster skin, fatigue, and more than you care to know.

No doubt, the subject of food, one's relationship with it, and its connection to a healthy body is a heady one. But in order for your body to function well, it needs to be *fed well* and your mind in turn must be fueled with the right directives to do so. No small goal. "I used to eat the unhealthiest food imaginable: baby back ribs, crème brulée, bacon and mayo sandwiches, fried chicken..." says Tyra Banks. Now the busy model says, "I'm trying to think before I eat. One reason is because I want that six-pack. Another is because I want to be healthy," Banks concludes. The young actress cites a number of family diseases as causes for her stance as well. "I'm a Black woman so high blood pressure, heart attacks, diabetes, and stroke, run in my people's genes," she says and adds, "I know this so now it's time to be smart. It's time to start eating to live, instead of living to eat."

I think now more than ever, we are challenged on many levels to refute today's common practices when it comes to food and to strive to tap into our origins as *the* way to live and equally important, thrive. Moreover, having an understanding of your body and its needs requires that you approach food as fuel, in other words as a source that promotes your well-being, within and without. This kind of thinking requires focus and commitment. When you think about it, food today is *so* associated with the various desires a stressed society hungers to fulfill. Therefore savvy marketing execs see to it that our minds are constantly being fueled with messages that subliminally proclaim food as the answer. Why who would believe the suggestion of a steamy, buttery roll accompanied by soft sounds, and a voiceover loaded with delicious adjectives isn't comforting? And when every other television commercial calls you to yet another mouth-watering delight—fast, frozen or otherwise—as an experience not to be missed, who among us wouldn't aim for it? Moreover, in a world where sugary soft drinks are associated with fun and success and those that are alcoholic promise pleasures untold, it's hard to imagine otherwise if you don't focus on the fine print—the things that aren't proclaimed. Truth is, the way food is cast today, it takes more than a notion to aim for that which is healthy, let alone not turn to it to satisfy our emotions or taste buds. According to Therman Evans, whose consulting firm, Whole Life Associates, is aimed at helping individuals maximize their potential and get the most out of life, "good-tasting food gives us a good feeling and we all love good feelings—the challenge is that all feelings, good and bad, have consequences. Unfortunately, we can have a good time feeling good headed straight to obesity, headed straight to heart disease, or arthritis that comes from carrying so much weight on the body," Evans concludes.

Another hurdle that throws many of us off track is that we tend to eat for taste as opposed to nutrition and the idea of what's *good* is usually those *fast* or processed foods that are chock-full of fat and sugar and more often than not, chemicals and dyes that impact our health. Holistic practitioners tell us to refute this practice by approaching food and the preparation of it as a very nurturing thing to do for ourselves. And as Evans asserts, aim for that which is more lasting and significant by putting an emphasis on eating a variety of God's natural offerings, like fresh fruits and vegetables. "Part of participating in your beauty is paying attention to the process, that's the kind of understanding that moves you to the point where you take charge because you know what facilitates your body on an intimate level," says Evans. Unfortunately, only a small percentage of us get the recommended servings per day of fruits and vegetables so key to a well body. However, as Tianuru points out, raw foods are like the body's cosmetics, enhancing both your inner and outer beauty. Eating for taste also causes us to tap into preparing our favorite foods in ways that aren't conducive to what's in the best interest of our health at times, such as frying over baking or broiling or adding smoked, carcinogenic meats to otherwise healthy dishes such as collard greens or lima beans. But experts say it's no wonder, given the history of people of African

It is a known fact that more than 90 percent of those who diet gain back every pound they lose and in some cases exceed their prediet weight. This proves that temporary plans come up short if for no other reason than the fact that the body cannot be sustained by such restrictions over a long period of time. In reality, achieving any physical goal comes by way of a focused mindset—based on a *lifestyle* change as opposed to that which is short term. Recent studies have evidenced that each person inherits a range of weights that his or her body can comfortably maintain, indicating that a person's weight range varies about 10 percent from a standard point. In other words, a 150-pound woman for example, might be able to weigh from 135 to 165, but every time her body dips below 135 or creeps beyond 165, her body will institute controls like an insatiable urge to eat more food or to consume less. The conclusion then according to the research is that one can keep their weight at the lower end of their range by watching what they eat and exercising.

As you and I know, being overweight ups the odds of developing heart disease, diabetes, increases your chances of having a stroke, and developing arthritis, so taking charge of this aspect of our lives is not a vain practice but a wise one. Most of all, make it a point to educate yourself about optimum health and fitness as opposed to thinness. Here are some simple guidelines to help you reach your goals:

- Slow your pace—it takes approximately twenty minutes for your brain to receive the proper signals that indicate you're full. So chew your food slowly and thoroughly and you'll find yourself satisfied, without a tendency to overeat.

- Don't skip breakfast—it breaks your fast and is essential to keeping your metabolism boosted.

- Don't go to extremes—a diet that cuts carbs or any other food group will make you more likely to later crave the same.

- Do make sure you get enough protein, which slows the movement of food, making you feel full longer.

- Watch your portions—in general, a single serving should be about the size of your palm.

descent here in the United States. "We as African people have been removed from our original state of being as fruitarians and vegetarians who ate very little meat on the Continent and have been asked to adapt to someone else's way of life," says Tianuru. Now, you and I know the *why* behind many of the traditional foods we eat: Our ancestors on these shores creatively put together the *leftovers* in order to survive. Today, that's no longer our truth. What's also no longer true is the nature of the foods they were accustomed to eating. Tianuru, who's also an iridologist and an herbalist, reminds us "the food that is being consumed now is not like that of our grandparents whose animals were free-ranged. They're being

- Eat carefully—your choices indicate the way you want to treat yourself. Resolve, then, to eat only the most nutritious foods.

- Pinpoint potential trouble spots like parties and come up with a strategy for coping such as eating a small, healthy meal at home beforehand so you won't arrive hungry, and then steer for only the healthiest choices while there—and drink lots of water.

- Don't bring temptation home—stock your fridge with smart choices and remember: "Faux foods," like those chock-full of sugar, artificial coloring, and chemicals are best left out!

- Don't fuel fatigue or depression—avoid sugar and caffeine, two culprits that also intensify cravings.

- Consume small healthy meals, rather than three big ones. This is the best way to burn fat, increase energy, and stave off cravings for snacks and sweets.

- Fend off cravings with healthy choices like water-rich fruits and raw veggies that'll help you to feel full. Look to apples, watermelon, celery, cucumbers, grapefruit, and grapes.

- Tend your emotional health by taking time for self—overdoing is not only stressful, but can lead to emotional eating, so don't take on too much.

- Stay spiritually connected—studies have shown a link between tending one's spirituality and sustained joy.

- Make sure you get the proper amount of exercise.

- Don't let yourself go—your appearance will affect how you feel about yourself as well as how you nurture your body, so strive to stay on track. If you overeat, make it a point to get right back in step with your goals .

- Get your rest! Lack of sleep not only compromises your mood and stimulates cravings, but impacts your immunity as well as your ability to exercise and recover.

- Stay positive—appreciate all that you are and be patient: Reaching your goals is both and inner and an outer process, and with diligence and focused work, you'll get to the finish line.

injected with hormones," she concludes. In fact, at the Afrikan Center of Well Being, clients are encouraged to eat *only* free-range protein and according Tia-nuru they come back happy to report that they feel better, both physically as well as emotionally. Moreover, as part of its mission to inform, the Center has educated many infertile couples by helping them to clean up their bodies and Tia-nuru says with an infectious joy, "they now have babies!" So many times we think things aren't within our control, but we've been programmed to give the control away. Now we have to take it back and utilize the power within and the best resources to have a quality of life that's wholesome and fulfilling.

Truth be told, tradition is hard to break, and so many things from our emotions to mental conditioning to outside stimulation fuel what we eat, but we need to prioritize our health and beauty and do that which will serve our highest good. In turn, we will always reap the best. So the wise path then is one of discipline, or "harnessing our power," as Tiranuru says, which simplifies one's life and creates balance.

To get on point, begin by giving reasonable focus to the kinds as well as the amount of food you consume. You might try recording your choices in a journal and making healthy substitutes for those foods that take more than they give. Be sure to look carefully at what you affirm on a daily basis as your mental aspect is the most important element to making behavioral modifications. Then take the stance that you are a cocreator in your life as Tianuru suggests and be determined to map out and adhere to what will cause you to thrive. To help strike a healthy balance, why not get better informed and begin by consulting a nutritionist or a holistic health care expert? Getting knowledgeable, professional advice is the soundest way to make sure that your eating plan is one that includes those foods (and food groups), as well as practical preparation methods, conducive to optimal health and beauty.

Supplemental Values

Shopping for vitamins these days can be a real trip—talk about hope in a jar! It doesn't get any bigger than this! With names like "Mega," "Super Potency," and "Stress Formula" and claims addressing everything from hair growth to weight loss, who can be totally certain how and what to choose to support their health? These are good reasons to become supplement-savvy so that you purchase only those that support basic bodily requirements, as well as any that provide for your unique needs. The supplements I take are guided by those on my temple management team, with particular input from my medical doctors and my iridologist. This is a very important part of taking care of my inner and outer beauty, and I rely on their knowledge and expertise as based on my exams to determine what's best for me. In general, I'm a pretty healthy eater, and I make sure to get a fresh vitamin and mineral boost from juicing vegetables and fruits, as well as incorporating ground flaxseed—rich in omega-3 fatty acids—into my favorite cereals, such as oatmeal. There are times, however, when anemia rears its head and I have to include an iron supplement. I don't smoke or drink alcoholic beverages, I consume few or no dairy products, and I'm pretty consistent at working out a minimum of three times a week. However, this is all in the face of long workdays, lots of air travel, and mornings savoring a half cup of coffee (albeit mostly decaf), all of which deplete vitamin stores and have a stressful impact on my body. Add to the equation the fact that women in my family are prone to benign cysts. Now here's a look at my supplement regimen at this point in my life and what it means:

- Multivitamin-mineral supplement daily—to provide the basic essentials

- 1,000 mg vitamin C daily when traveling—to boost the immune system and counteract the negative effects of crossing time zones

- 400 mg vitamin E daily—to address cysts, serve as an immune booster

- Chlorophyll daily—to promote blood and colon health

- Acidophilus three times a week—to provide healthy bacteria (in the intestinal system in the absence of eating foods such as yogurt, which are a good source)

- 1,000 mg calcium citrate daily—to protect against bone loss (calcium citrate is more easily absorbed by the body than other forms of calcium)

I share my profile with you as a good way to highlight the value of trusting the selection of supplements that are right for you to the pros and not going at this as a solo act. I could never have judged my need for the above on my own, or the fact that my coffee intake was preventing the absorption of nutrients. (Now there's a real reason to quit drinking it!) The supplements we take should always be based on our health, age, lifestyle, and diet. How do you ascertain whether or not you need a multivitamin with iron unless your blood test and your health care professional indicate that you need one? Or how can you determine when it's safe to go beyond the RDA requirements for any vitamin? Or if the source of your iron is the proper one for you? The risks of error are far too great for you to leave this aspect of your health and beauty to generalizations and chance. Supplements play a very valuable role in helping us support ourselves when combined with a healthy eating plan. On a fundamental level, you do need those that are essential for development, to support your immune system, to help convert food to energy, and to support your unique needs—everything else is best left on the shelf.

The Essential Role of Water

I was never big on water until I came of age and learned that it is essential to life. I cringe when I think about all the years I passed up on its benefits in lieu of soft drinks, and I know I often didn't realize I was dehydrated and turned instead to

Supporting your body from within with the healthiest foods and targeted supplements that meet your needs and desires is crucial in this day and age. The right supplements play an all-important role in every aspect of your beauty, from your internal health and well-being to the integrity of your hair, skin, and nails. Most experts will recommend a multivitamin and multimineral formula, supplemented by calcium and magnesium. Today, many health-care practitioners will also include herbs in your personal roundup to provide additional support and address specific needs. Just remember, to get the most from your supplements, take them with food, since fat aids the absorption of nutrients, and always store them in a cool, dark place, as sunlight can decrease their potency. Here is a list of the basics the experts deem necessary to support one's health and beauty:

Vitamin A – an antioxidant, promotes skin health, enhances immunity

B Complex (thiamine, riboflavin, niacin, pantothenic acid, pyridoxine, cyanocobalamin, biotin, choline, folate, inositol)—anti-stress, energy boosting, enhances circulation, cell growth, healthy hair

Vitamin C – an antioxidant, promotes the production of collagen; helps boost the immune system and healthy gums, increases the absorption of iron

Vitamin D – essential to the proper absorption of calcium, essential for growth, strong bones, and healthy teeth

Vitamin E – an antioxidant; protects skin from oxidative damage; improves the immune system, circulation, useful in treating fibrocystic breasts

MINERALS:

Calcium – helps prevent bone loss, builds strong teeth, healthy gums

Chromium – energy boosting, maintains stable blood sugar levels

Copper – aids in the formation of bones, red blood cells, promotes healthy nerves and joints

Magnesium – usually combined with calcium, supports nerve and muscle function

Potassium – promotes a healthy nervous system, aids in proper muscle contraction

Selenium – enhances the absorption of vitamin E, protects the immune system

Zinc – promotes tissue and cell growth, healthy immune system, bone formation

food or over-the-counter medicines in an attempt to relieve headaches and other unexplainable symptoms. "Most of the cellular content of our bodies is water. When we don't have enough of it we have all kinds of problems, from constipation to headaches, dizziness, poor memory, poor concentration, and fatigue," says Dr. Andrea Sullivan. "Any one of those symptoms can be a result of not having enough water and being dehydrated." Furthermore, when you're dehydrated, your body holds on to fluid, making you look puffy. Many of us are afraid to consume too much water because of bloating, but in fact it's excess salt intake and too many carbs that contribute to this, not water.

According to the experts, a *minimum* of six to eight glasses daily is essential just to help the body function properly. But many other factors figure into why *you* may need far more than this—from whether or not you work out or drink coffee, tea, or other caffeinated beverages (caffeine is dehydrating) to whether or not it's hot and humid out, what altitude you live at, or if you simply have a common cold. These and other aspects call for you to drink up way beyond the minimum.

Water is responsible for such life-sustaining functions as:

- Regulating body temperature

- Transporting nutrients

- Eliminating wastes

- Dissolving many vitamins and minerals

- Providing a liquid cushion for the brain and spinal cord

Water also hydrates skin cells and keeps them plump. Moreover, consuming enough water is unbeatable for regularity. "If one was to drink four or five glasses of water in the morning when they get up, they'd have regular bowel movements," says Dr. Therman Evans.

For some of us, water is an acquired taste—in other words, we just don't care for it plain and simple. My mother was in that category, and for a long time so was I. I had become conditioned to satisfying my taste buds, and so anything sweet was, in my mind, the thirst quencher that had my name on it. Needless to say, I allowed *taste* to govern this aspect of my life as opposed to letting wisdom rule. But watching my mother struggle with kidney disease taught me some powerful lessons about what to help myself to and what to turn away from. So I can't urge you enough to put down the coffee, tea, and colas and reach for water every chance you get, if for no other reason than this sobering news from Dr. Sullivan:

"When you start fooling around with caffeine, you get into fibroid territory. Fibroids love all the things that have caffeine—tea, coffee, anything caffeinated," she concludes. We know all too well that an overwhelmingly large number of us suffer with fibroids. In a recent study by the National Institute of Environmental Health Sciences conducted on more than a thousand women between the ages of 35 and 49, 72 percent of those who were African-Americans had fibroids. So let's drink to our health and make getting enough water a priority. All it takes is persistence and a deep desire to do what's best for you. For me, water has become my best accessory—I carry it with me all the time!

To find a naturopath in your area, contact the following:

The American Association of Naturopathic Physicians
(877) 969-2267 or www.naturopathic.org

The California Association of Naturopathic Physicians
(800) 521-1200 or www.canp.org

The American Naturopathic Medical Association
(702) 897-7053 or www.anma.com

Washington Association of Naturopathic Physicians
(206) 547-2130 or www.wanp.org

To find an Ayurvedic Practitioner, contact the following:

American Holistic Health Association
(714) 779-6152 or www.ahha.org

California Association of Ayurvedic Medicine
(800) 292-4882 or www.ayurveda-caam.org

SELF-SEDUCTION

PARTNERING WITH A NUTRITIONIST

Consulting a nutritionist is like working with a guide on a new adventure. During my first experience I was swept away in one session by the knowledge I gained about certain foods and how I could reach a variety of my goals through the proper combinations—and deletions! Says Oz Garcia, nutritional consultant to such A-listers as model Veronica Webb and actress Sanaa Lathan, "Today when women think about food, they need to think in terms of: What does it take to regulate your hormones? Your appearance in ways that promote stability and a healthy state of mind? What food gives you a stronger brain? Makes you less prone to PMS?" This kind of thinking represents a criterion for a new day. I know I never thought of food in this way, but reaching our best selves now and in the future clearly will require the kind of examination as well as discipline that Garcia is suggesting. Garcia, who has authored two bestsellers, *The Balance* and *The Healthy High Tech Body*, believes a nutritionist "really helps one to be thoughtful when it comes to food." Webb, who's benefited from his sage advice for the last ten years (which no doubt has given her an edge in a highly competitive career), says she's learned that restricting herself a little every day is easier than going up and down on crash diets. "I've developed a discipline to stop eating when I'm full, and certain things I try not to eat at all—wheat, sugar, dairy—as my body doesn't process that stuff really well," says the busy model.

In preparation for visits with a nutritionist, whether locally or anytime I have the opportunity to see one at a spa, I've learned to jot down what I want to accomplish and reminders about what I want to ask: which foods will help me maintain my weight and increase energy, to ask alternatives to sweets, ways to handle less-than-healthy cravings, how to satisfy the yearning for certain textures (I love foods with that crunch factor, but don't want all that fat and sodium that usually accompanies them). More and more, I'm learning how to avoid sugar in all its disguises and what to consume to stave off illness, especially those that are prevalent in my family, like heart disease and stroke. Most of all, like many women in the know, I've learned how valuable it is to have a nutritionist as part of my temple management team to ensure a better me.

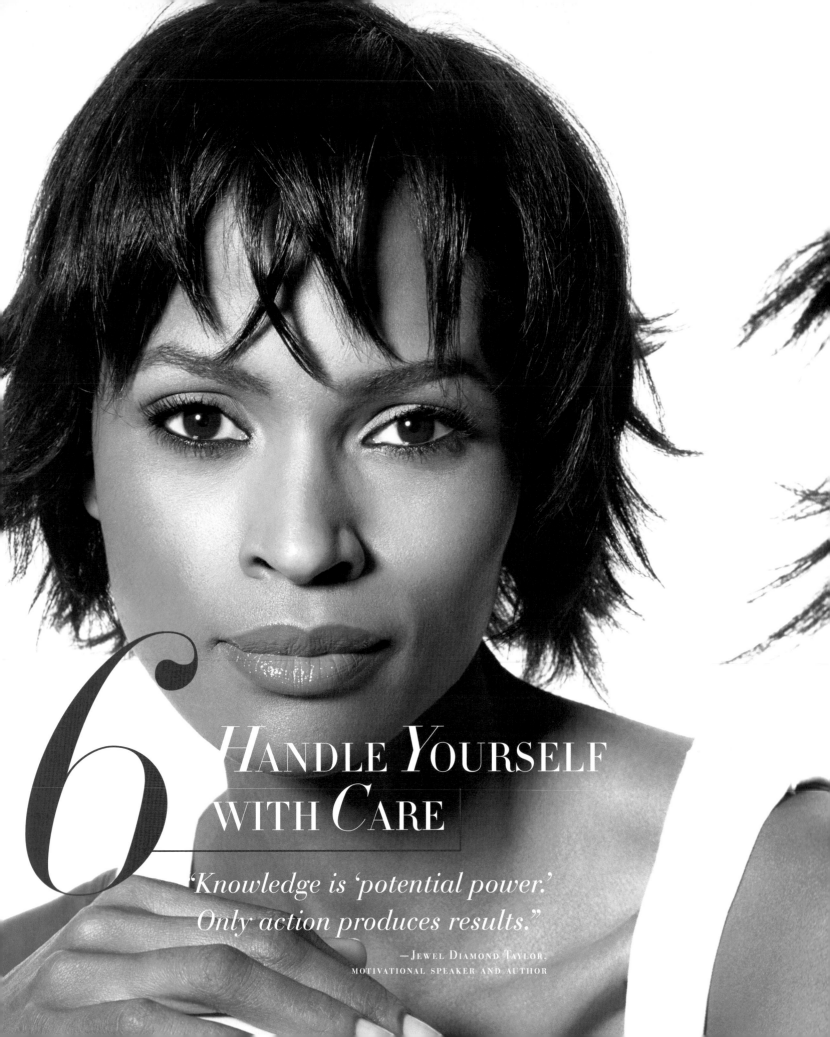

6 HANDLE YOURSELF WITH CARE

"Knowledge is 'potential power.'
Only action produces results."

—JEWEL DIAMOND TAYLOR,
MOTIVATIONAL SPEAKER AND AUTHOR

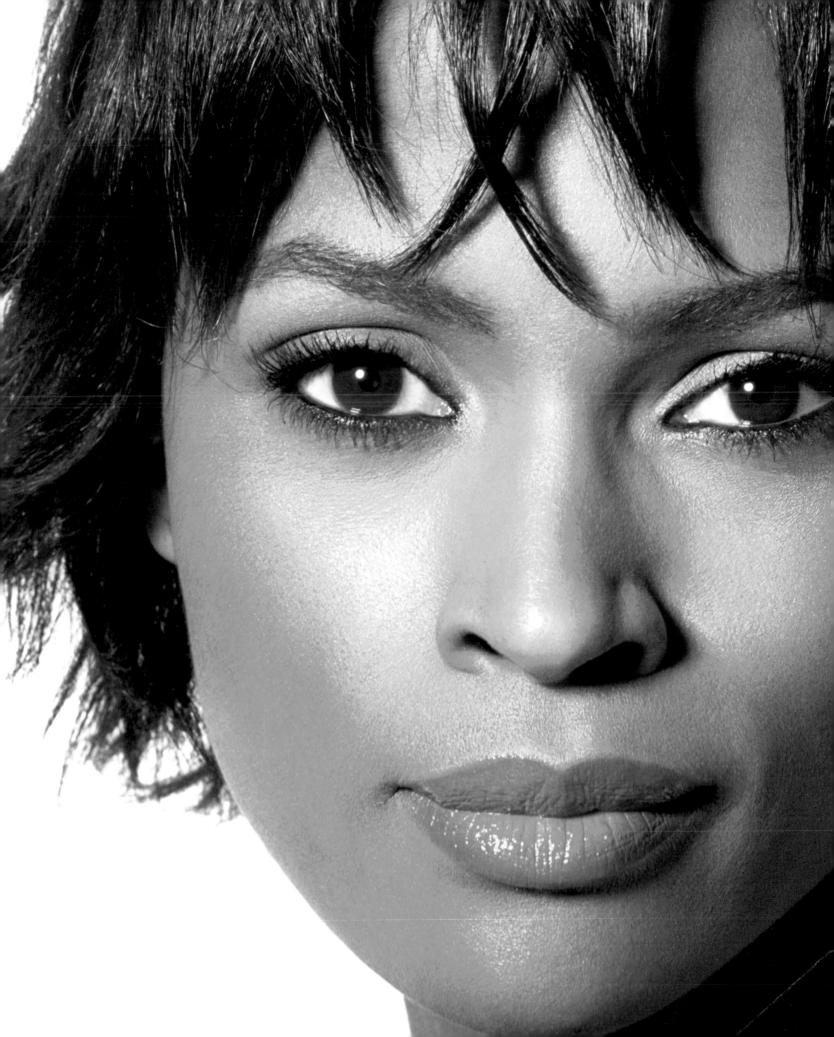

Years ago there was a hilarious play on Broadway called *Stop the World—I Want to Get Off.* And let me tell you, there was a time in my life when I could really relate. I had gotten to the point where I felt like I just couldn't keep up. Life had become a one-woman show that could easily have been entitled *Hurry Up, Girlfriend!* And believe it or not, I had the rhythm and was starring in the show, until one day I fell while rushing up the stairs trying to do my minimum of two things at once and did some real damage. Due to my haste, I ended up taking on yet another responsibility, that of learning how to control two friends who were going to assist me for a while: a pair of crutches! That's when I realized that the show had to stop, because for one thing, I recognized that I had no stand-in. For another, I was tired of the pace—and not only the one that was obviously self-imposed, but the general fast-forward pace I continue to feel around me, which has altered the way we treat ourselves and caused us to hurry through life taking ourselves for granted.

Quite frankly, we live in a world that values people who can multitask. It's easy to see how we've become comfortable accomplishing the more-than-formidable. In fact, this is true not only at large, but even among ourselves—we have a tendency to high-five those who can move the world in a day. More often than not, we encourage one another in this behalf with a "go on, girl" send-off. "We want to go twenty-four/seven, and yet there is no other species in this world that goes at it like humans," says Pamela J. Peters, Ph.D., president and founder of the Center for Stress, Pain, and Wellness Management in Wilmington, Delaware. Unfortu-

SELF-SEDUCTION

nately, we don't realize that there's a high price on those pearls of accomplishment. That in and of itself is so hard to come to terms with because we grew up in this mode. Our mothers, grandmothers, and those who kept watch over us were up before the sun, turning the world and pushing us to get on with it and conduct ourselves in a like manner. So the very idea of handling ourselves with care was almost foreign, because we grew up thinking that care was something you gave to someone else. So now here we are in the fullness of our womanhood, in arrival time, just beginning to get the lesson. And it shows up in ways that we don't even question and causes us to gauge everything in terms of efficiency. As a result, we end up with one ear on our children and the other on the phone, or touching up our nails in the car each time we stop at a red light rather than in the privacy of our homes. We hit the shower as if we're passing through the car wash and then slap on a little lotion, instead of taking the time for a bath and the appreciation of our own gentle touch. And every day we go at our lives in run-run-run mode, instead of aligning our thinking in a way that allows us to move at a reasonable pace and handle ourselves with care. We also ignore the little warning signs that tell us to go easy or stop moving too fast, until something dramatic happens, and then we're forced to treat ourselves differently, reevaluating our strengths and how we utilize our energy. Model Karen Alexander had one of those happenings several years ago—it compromised her health to the point where her legs became incredibly weak, almost paralyzed. After months of medical testing, including an MRI and a spinal tap that ruled out multiple sclerosis, the busy model, who was recognized as one of *People* magazine's "50 Most Beautiful People," said she took that time of being flat on her back to do a life review and finally understood that it was okay not to be going and doing all the time. Now she goes about life at her own pace, balancing work with a particular emphasis on raising daughters Zora and Ella well. This she does by reminding herself of that "tell-all" moment in life, spending more quality time with them, and taking care of herself. She says, "That part of my life taught me that I had to make things simple in all parts of my life and operate differently, and treat *myself* in the way I would treat anyone that I love." No stranger to accolades, actress Halle Berry has earned the finest, from the coveted Emmy and Golden Globe, to that which dreams are made of, the Oscar. Nevertheless, the softspoken actress recalls there was a time when she had to learn the importance of honoring oneself and the kind of care that goes along with it. "During my twenties, I was really hard on myself, really judgmental, and expected way too much of myself, and in some ways that served me well, but in other ways it was really destructive, because I found myself being insecure about who I was and not realizing my own value and my own worth. Instead I was constantly putting myself down, not being gentle and affirming with myself, but allowing what other people thought of me to be my view of me. When I got to around thirty, something in me shifted and I thought hmmm, this isn't quite working, relying on other people to be easy with me because nobody was and I learned that I have to be gentle and easy with me and take care of me and love myself and not rely on other people to," she said.

Actress LaTanya Richardson Jackson, whose moving portrayals of strong, independent women caused her to land roles on cable television's A&E drama *100 Centre Street* and HBO's *Introducing Dorothy Dandridge*, says she too has only begun to handle herself with care, because prior to this period in her life she never thought she needed to. The bicoastal Jackson, who spends her time balancing family life and career, said that while growing up she made herself very strong because her mother was gone a lot and she had to deal with that. "I was trying to be the strong one all the time, so I never thought I needed to be handled with care. I made myself a nurturer of others and told myself, 'I'm fine, I can get through it no matter what,'" she confesses. Jackson says she recently realized she was at a point where she'd done that for so long that she felt herself breaking. Her turnaround came with the realization that loving yourself isn't just a statement, nor is it about covering up your needs; rather, it's about taking action and listening to all of *you*. So these days you'll find her "taking greater care listening to my body and myself, and seeing and addressing my needs," as she puts it. Like many of us, the actress says she never questioned why she was running and doing, nor the fact that she was tired. Now, however, she will often pause and say, "Wait a minute—I *am* tired, so maybe I'm not going to do this or that."

When you think about it, we've been given one unique vessel to honor and richly enjoy. Haste is contrary to these privileges. Furthermore, "when you're stressed trying to do ninety million things, what you're doing is giving a little bit of yourself with an attitude," says Peters, and that's a testimony we *don't* want to be true of us. We also need to do away with some of the things we've accepted as truth, especially that myth that makes us believe we can do it all and not injure ourself in the process. I watched my mother overwork herself going and doing for everyone else, and when it came time for her to retire, what ought to have been her glory days were spent in ill health. And although our paths are a lot different today, I recognize that if we're not careful, the same could easily be true of us. So, my sisters, I'm saying it's time for us to create a new script. I want something better for us and for those who'll follow in our stead. We have to begin by telling ourselves the truth and then living it out. Growing up, I waited what seemed like an eternity to enjoy the pleasures of being a woman. Being overwrought and too tired to be the woman I dreamed of becoming is not what I had in mind. Consequently, I'm committed to handling myself with care so that I can appreciate all of me. I'm learning not to enter myself in a contest for overachievers that I have no desire to win. I'm moving to that place where I say no to those things that I don't need to be doing. And like LaTanya and many of you who have reached this realization already, I'm so much better for it. In particular, I've learned to take good care of my feet and hands—the parts of me that are always running and doing. For example, the corns on my toes are disappearing because I'm not trying to "break in" shoes that don't fit. I'm not clenching my fists over stressful occurrences. I'm not cutting my cuticles, because I know they're there not to satisfy my vanity but to protect my body from infection. And speaking of protection, I've learned to take that extra step by bringing a bag with my personal manicure tools along with me when having a professional manicure, because I know from the experts that utensils shouldn't be shared with strangers due to bacteria and transmissible infections.

Most of all, I make sure to keep my hands and feet well groomed, because this not only makes me feel good but says to the outside world that I value every aspect of my beauty, from head to toe. Ditto for what I put in my body, especially those good things like lots of protein, calcium, and fruits and vegetables to fortify my temple and keep my skin and nails healthy and strong. You know, handling yourself with care isn't about being self-indulgent, and it certainly doesn't mean acting like a princess or a diva. It simply comes down to making wise choices and turning some of the care that we know how to give so well back on ourselves.

Essential Nail Tools

The secret to a great manicure can be summed up in a word: quality! And everything from the amount of time you give yourself and your frame of mind to the type of products and tools you choose to use should be hinged on this to ensure not only that you achieve the most beautiful results but that it becomes a pampering experience as well. From this perspective, caring for your nails is simply another way of honoring yourself. As you prepare for this restorative ritual, equip yourself with the best tools and pampering treats your money can buy. Here's an overall checklist of the supplies that'll help you nail it for sure:

- Nail brush

- Small bowl

- Emery board

- Buffing disc

- Pumice stick

- Orangewood stick

- Loose cotton

- Acetone-free polish remover

- Cuticle remover or softener

- Body scrub

- Shower gel

- Hand towel

- Hand cream

- Base coat and topcoat

- Polish

A Perfect 10

Giving back to yourself through a manicure is a treat that takes so little time but gives so much in return, from the joy that accompanies self-nurturing to the empowerment of personal reflection. So look forward to this time and take it to another level by penciling it in on your weekly schedule, preparing for it with the right tools, and selecting a special place in your home that beckons you to quiet and calm. Trust me, you don't want to care for yourself in front of the television set or while trying to perform another task at the same time—this isn't the time to try to kill two birds with one stone! Know that you deserve better and commit to it as a time you devote to yourself, uninterrupted and without distraction, unless of course you have a daughter or a special sister friend in your life for whom this experience will enhance a shared sacred space and serve as an example of guilt-free nurturing. Once you're ready to begin, follow this route to a perfect 10:

- Begin by massaging hands with a creamy body scrub. Then wash hands thoroughly with the shower gel and pat dry.

- Saturate a small portion of loose cotton—much more absorbent than cotton balls—with polish remover and remove all polish from your nails.

- File nails gently, in one direction, into your preferred shape. "Do not saw your nails back and forth," says manicurist Von Christmas, of Le Skintique Salon, located in Englewood, California, as doing so will weaken them. Follow by using the buffing disc lightly on the edges and to smooth any rough areas on the surface of the nail.

Model
Nichole Robinson

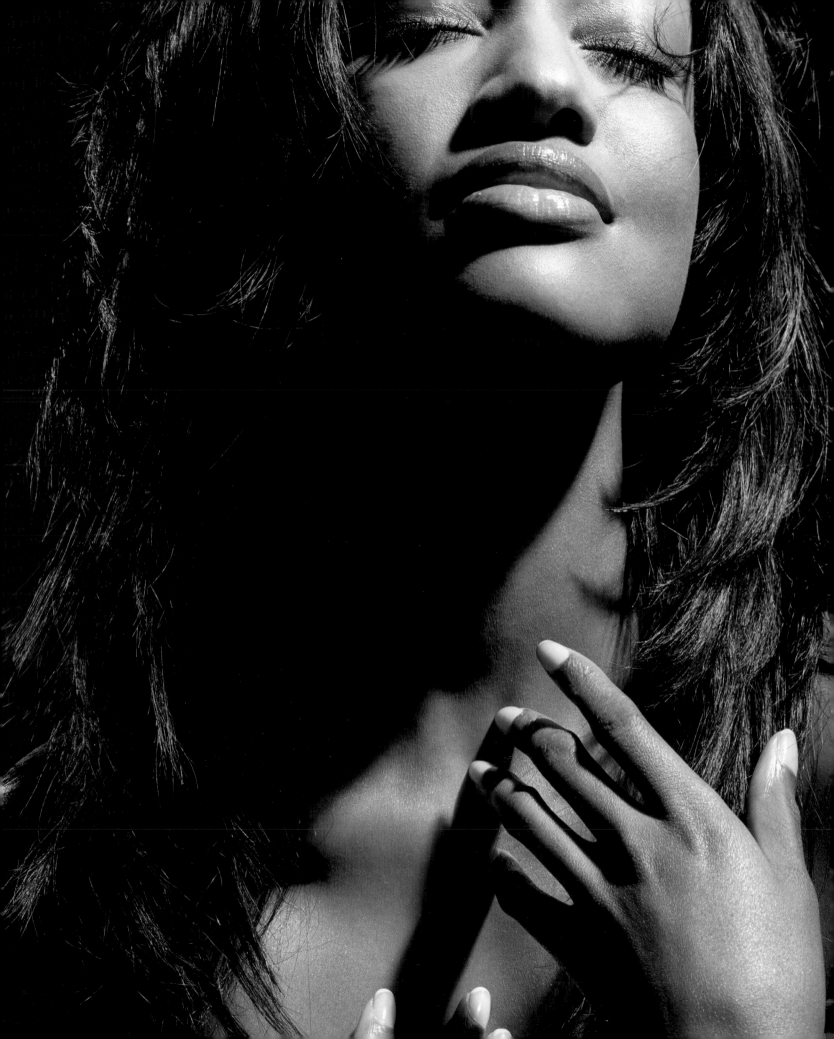

MAXIMIZE YOUR MANICURE

Needless to say, when it comes to color and style, we delight in taking this ritual of beautifying ourselves to an art form. However, be aware that everything from the condition of your nails to the wearing of tips and acrylic extensions, from daily personal maintenance to how you live your life, will impact your manicure and how long it will last. To help you prolong yours, here are a few tips from the pros:

- Condition your nails by hydrating them at every opportunity to keep them healthy and resilient. Do so by massaging oil onto both the nails and your cuticles. Excellent choices, according to Tamika Hardy of Come to You, which services busy executives in the New York City area with in-office hand and foot treatments, are jojoba, sweet almond, and avocado. Regular application of oil not only hydrates your cuticles and your nails, says Hardy, but it also keeps your polish from chipping, which happens because water dries it out, so when you hydrate your nails, you hydrate the polish as well. Overall, try to follow the advice of Julie Serquinia of the Paint Shop in Beverly Hills, who says the best way to prolong your manicure is to treat your nails as though you just got them polished. Simply put, that means taking special care with them every day, from the way you pick things up to not using them as tools.

- Protect your polish by "wearing rubber gloves when doing household duties and by applying a topcoat every three days," says manicurist Von Christmas. And always make sure to cover the tips, where polish begins to chip due to daily activities. If you wear acrylics, your manicurist should use a bonder base—a rubberized formula that allows the polish to adhere to the nail base, according to Cyndi Watson, of L.A.'s Millennium Salon. "Then follow up every other day with topcoat," says the busy nail technician, who travels on set to give Queen Latifah a perfect 10.

- Experts concur that the surface of the nail also has a lot to do with how long your polish will last. New York manicurist Deborah Lippman advises using a ridge-filler base coat, as it has fibers and polish will adhere to the nails better. Bernadette Thompson, of the Tips-n-Toes Salon in New York City, who ensures a perfect 10 for Mary J. Blige and Missy Elliott, finds that buffing the nails but not making them too smooth helps, as the polish has something to hold on to; she cites this as a reason why polish rarely chips off acrylic nails, as they're not really smooth.

- How polish is applied also plays a role. Here it's best to think thin and allow polish to dry between coats—"two minutes," says Lippman. And she adds, "Make sure to swipe the brush across the tip of the nails," which take the most wear and tear in between manicures.

- Alcohol is a big culprit when it comes to compromising the longevity of your manicure, as it strips away your polish and dries your nails. Since it's found in many beauty goods that we use on a daily basis, take care to avoid contact with the nails when using products in which it is contained, such as hair gels and holding sprays.

- Finally, skip the use of quick-dry topcoats, which, according to Lippman, shrink nail polish as they dry, making polish chip faster.

- Apply cuticle softener and soak hands in warm water, along with any additions you like to use. Christmas in particular likes to add an effervescent hand sanitizer, available at most beauty supply stores, as it softens the cuticles. However, if your nails are weak, New York City–based manicurist S. Michele Echols, who paints a perfect 10 for singer Ashanti, urges you to skip soaking your nails in water, which she says can wear down the nail plate, and simply wash your hands after pushing back your cuticles.

- Using the nail brush, gently cleanse the nails on top and underneath and pat dry.

- Gently push back your cuticles with the pumice stick.

- Apply hand cream and take just a moment to massage your hands, from the inside of the wrist to your palms and on to the back of your hands and fingers. If you have very dry hands and nails, try the hydrating heat treatment featured for the feet. You can also invest in a paraffin heater, which is superb for this purpose.

- Now you're ready for polish. Begin by cleaning the nail surface, using cotton and the orangewood stick, with a bit of remover; also clean under the tip. Apply base coat to the nails starting at the bottom center of the nail bed and extending to the tip. Repeat to complete the entire nail and allow it to dry. Then apply two coats of polish, allowing for some drying time in between. Using the orangewood stick, remove any excess polish that may have seeped into the cuticles or onto your skin. Then apply the topcoat and allow it to dry completely.

Trouble Spots

Let's face it—despite our best efforts, modern life has a way of impacting our beauty, particularly those areas that are always on display, like our nails. When you couple that with the things that are tough to control, such as the effects of aging and environmental exposure, you recognize that maintaining your nails requires a proactive strategy to keep them pretty and problem-free. What also helps is knowing how to resolve troublesome concerns as they arise, with these maneuvers from the pros:

CHIPS The idea is to prep the surface of the area where polish has chipped, therefore making it easy to repair. To do so, Lippmann suggests you "wet the pad of a finger using nail polish remover and lightly dab it on the chip to smooth it down (hint: brush from where the chip begins, out toward the tip of the nail) and let it dry. Then dab your polish there, allow it to dry for about thirty seconds, then brush the whole nail with the color." Finish with a shiny topcoat to seal the deal. Also, never use remover to thin out thickened polish, as it will weaken the formula, causing it to chip easily—instead, use a polish thinner.

DISCOLORATIONS According to Dr. Richard Scher, professor of dermatology and a nail specialist at Columbia University in New York City, discoloration can be the result of a number of circumstances, including trauma, certain medications, bacterial or fungus infections, or diabetes. "If the discoloration is brown, it could be due to antibiotics; if one nail is brown, however, it could be melanin and probably should be checked by a dermatologist," he says. "Most white spots are due to trauma, i.e., having your cuticles pushed back so vigorously that the matrix (the nail growth center) is injured." His prescription: be gentle, skip the use of metal and wooden instruments, soak the cuticles in warm water, and push them back using a moist towel or washcloth. If areas of green begin to appear, that's a sure indication of a bacterial infection, whereas yellow, according to Scher, can indicate a fungus infection (a yellow color occurs more commonly in diabetics as well). It's best to see a dermatologist for proper diagnosis, who can best determine a follow-up; if infection is present, this may include oral or topical medications. Yellowing of the nails can also come from prolonged wearing of dark polish, particularly without a base coat, in which case Hardy advises the use of lemon juice to whiten the nails and cancel out the dye that has been absorbed by the nail from the polish.

PEELING NAILS Peeling signals a loss of moisture and calls for consistent hydration. Thompson offers this restorative advice: "Heat a cup of olive oil in the microwave for ten seconds and soak your nails in it." She also strongly advises sisters with dry nails to forgo soaking their nails in water, particularly during the winter months. Instead, she says, substitute warm lotion. Using an appropriate strengthener will also help put you on the road to recovery. Prevention plays a role in strengthening nails prone to peeling as well—aside from a healthy diet and the use of moisturizers, Scher cautions us to avoid products that are drying, such as nail polish removers that contain acetone and polish that isn't formaldehyde- and toluene-free.

BRITTLE NAILS Genetics, excess exposure to water, and a lack of calcium can cause nails to become brittle and break. Consulting your doctor about calcium supplements and increasing the intake of this mineral from rich sources such as milk, yogurt, sardines, and salmon can help, as can incorporating the use of a nail strengthener and a hydrating oil. Making sure to avoid the use of products that are drying and wearing rubber gloves as much as possible when nails are exposed to cleaning agents and water will also make a difference. You might also look for lotions containing alpha-acetoxy acid, said to prevent brittleness and control peeling.

RIDGES Nail ridges are basically a by-product of the aging process, although according to Scher they can happen to the young as well. They can also be accentuated by overexposure to the sun. "Nails are subject to sun damage just like the skin is," Scher informs us. Manicurist Tamika Hardy says the simplest strategy is to buff the nails lightly, use a ridge-filler base coat to give nails a smooth and lustrous appearance, and avoid the use of sheer nail lacquers, sticking to creams instead.

SPLITTING CUTICLES Very dry skin and excessive picking and/or cutting contribute to this condition. To avoid, treat cuticles with the TLC they deserve and pamper them by massaging cuticle oil onto them a few times a day. To heal, I've found a combination of tea tree oil and vitamin E, which can be found in a health food store, works wonders! Ditto for petroleum jelly or an over-the-counter antibiotic ointment, applied at night when hands are at rest, especially if used in conjunction with cotton gloves (if the splitting is confined to just a few nails, you can substitute a bandage for the gloves). If, however, you find that your cuticles become red, swollen, or tender, an infection may be present, in which case it's wise to see a dermatologist.

HANGNAILS According to Hardy, hangnails are a result of extremely dry skin, where the skin surrounding the nails becomes brittle and peels away. Treat by replenishing lost moisture with a good hand cream, preferably one that contains alpha-hydroxy acids, or cuticle oil. Always clip hangnails using a cuticle nipper— never pull them. "When you pull on a hangnail, you're actually ripping the skin and you put yourself at risk for soreness and infection," adds Hardy.

Sole Food

Today we live in an age where our feet and legs are likely to be on view all year long. I don't know whom we have to thank—fashion designers or our sister celebs who consistently hit the scene in the most sensuous footwear sans hose every time they step out. I remember the time when we didn't even think about such exposure until beach season rolled around. But now, sound self-care and the ability to live as we choose and not skip a beat inspires us to manage this aspect of our beauty year round. Keeping tootsies sandal-ready is no feat when you incorporate their care into your body-maintenance routine with a proven strategy that makes it simple and easy. To get started, here's what you need to have on hand:

- Foot file or pumice stone

- Emery boards

- Nail buffer

- Nail clippers

- Cotton swabs

- Basin

- Two small hand towels and one bath towel

- Toe separators

- Two large plastic bags

- Cuticle remover

- Hydrating foot cream

- Polish remover

- Polish

Now you're ready to begin your own deluxe pedicure. Make it count by selecting a quiet space where you can get comfortable, without interruption, for thirty to forty-five minutes. Set your sounds for complete relaxation, and perhaps enhance the experience with a soothing candle.

- Remove old polish using an acetone-free polish remover.

- Soak feet in warm water for approximately ten to fifteen minutes to soften cuticles, calluses, and rough skin. To enhance the experience, add a few drops of essential oil to the water (relaxing lavender or sage would be a good choice) and half a cup of milk to soften. Hardy also recommends adding sanitizing tea tree oil and a tablespoon of almond oil to hydrate. After the soaking phase, remove and pat dry.

- File, using a coarse emery board, or clip toenails straight across to prevent ingrown nails. Smooth edges with a fine emery board. Hit heels and calluses with a paddle-type foot file—preferably one that's fine-grained so that you're removing dead skin buildup and refining the texture of your feet at the same time, as opposed to roughing up the surface. This type of foot file instantly turns dry skin to dust, leaving a fine, smooth surface. Follow by applying a cuticle remover and then gently push the cuticles back. This is also a good time to buff the nails for smoothness.

SELF-SEDUCTION

Model
Rochelle Hunt

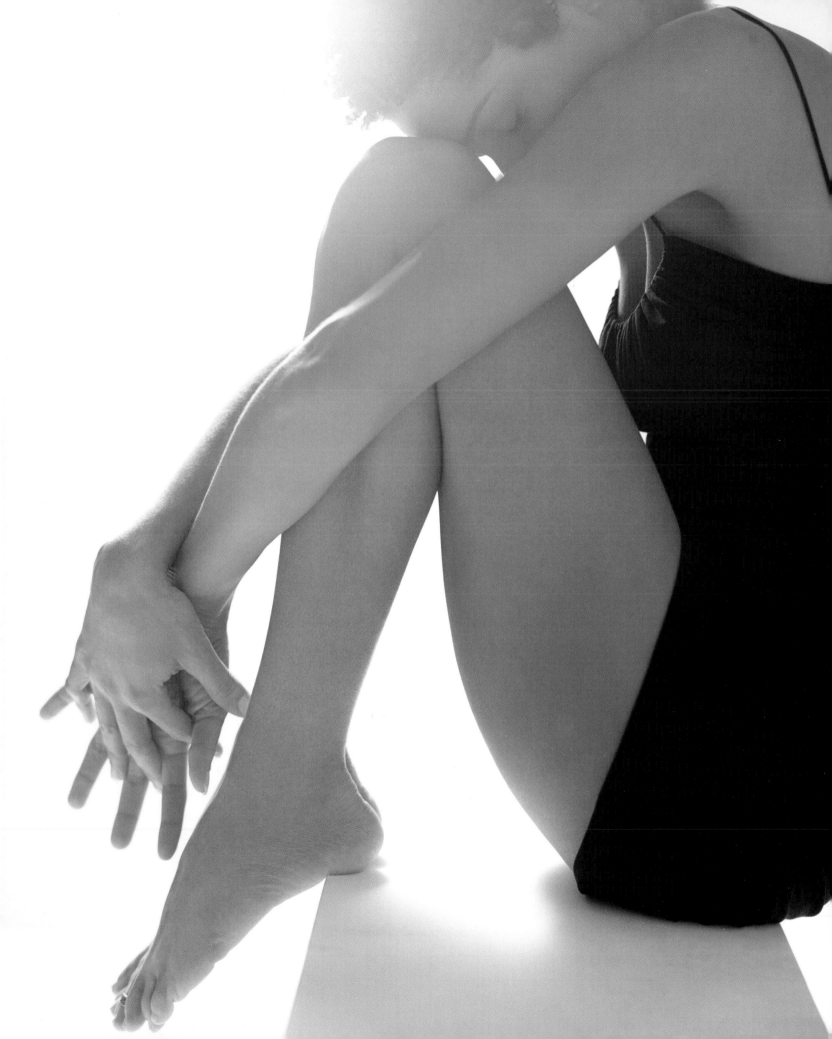

- Exfoliate feet all over using a palmful of body scrub, or make your own. I like to mix baby oil and sea salt (available at health food stores) to form a paste that further refines the skin, leaving feet kissably soft!

- Then treat feet to a hydrating mask by applying a rich foot cream. Lippman advises looking to those that contain shea butter, and perhaps some peppermint to aid with swelling, methylparaben to moisturize, and glycolic acid to take away dead skin. Follow this application by placing each foot into a plastic bag, wrapping a comfortably hot hand towel around each, and letting it remain on for five minutes for the heat and the moisture to penetrate. Remove plastic bags and massage any residue into skin. Put on your toe separators and give toes a once-over using a swab applicator dipped in polish remover to make sure the entire surface of each nail, "as well as the tip and underneath it, are really clean and dry," says Lippman.

- Now you're ready for polish. Whether you're going for a nice nude or a knockout color, follow the pros' advice to get professional results. "Always wipe off one side of the brush and use the *other* side to apply the polish, using light brush strokes," says Echols. And remember to use thin coats, which Lippman says dry better. Both will make for a smooth, even application of color. Begin with your preferred base coat, followed by two coats of polish and a topcoat.

Maintain satiny feet by applying a good foot cream, preferably one that contains skin-softening alpha-hydroxy acids, after your morning shower; at night, you can't beat good old petroleum jelly with a pair of socks or booties! Keep a foot file in the bathroom, where it'll be handy for biweekly touch-ups on heels and other areas of the foot where you may have a tendency to build up dead skin. And get comfortable pampering them day to day. Says Julie Serquinia, who cares for such high-profile clients as Nia Long and *Access Hollywood*'s Sean Robinson, "Regardless of what your budget is, there are things you can do, like go to the grocery store and buy safflower, canola, or olive oil, which can be used as a massage oil to make you feel good." No matter how tempted you may find yourself, never trim cuticles or use a razor to remove calluses or buildup. Cuticles should only be pushed back, and gently at that. As for using a razor, such serious maneuvers are best left to the pros. Corns are best treated by a podiatrist, who'll safely remove them using a method that's best for you. If the corn is severe, a surgical procedure that involves shaving it down to relieve the pressure may be called for. To prevent them from occurring, remember to give feet a break from high heels as often as possible and "pay attention to shoes that cramp your feet," adds Lippman. Truth

FANCY FEET

Well-cared-for feet and perfectly groomed nails are simple pleasures. The fun begins when you personalize a look with distinctive touches, whether in the form of a beguiling toe ring, a charming nail adornment, a discreet tattoo, or unexpected color. One way to have fun is with a French pedicure, which the pros say is here to stay. Here are a few of their favorite variations on this newly-coined classic, as well as some other savvy takes that'll help you put your best foot forward:

"Flip the French manicure by adding a nice gold or silver edge,
or adding a sheer shimmer overlay."
TAMIKA HARDY, COME TO YOU

"Stones always work, whether on a single toe or to emphasize
a French manicure!"
BERNADETTE THOMPSON, TIP-N-TOES SALON, NEW YORK CITY

"Try a matte coral with a hot, iridescent pink swiped across the tip,
or an opaque beige with a red tip—how sexy!"
DEBORAH LIPPMAN, NEW YORK CITY

"Try a soft blue with a slightly darker or lighter trim, or rhinestones!"
JULIE SERQUINIA, PAINT SHOP, BEVERLY HILLS

is, living in high heels not only damages your feet but can cause back and knee pain and really throw your posture off. And stilettos, particularly those of the pointed-toe variety, can cause hammertoes and bunions. Not very pretty! So be sure to rotate the type of shoes you wear as well as the heel height.

To keep stepping in style, it's a good idea to give yourself a pedicure every three to four weeks. You might also consider a *medical pedicure*, which is performed by podiatrist. These usually go the extra mile when it comes to care. During this procedure, the health of your feet is analyzed with follow-up care advice, corns and calluses are appropriately removed, and if necessary, perhaps a glycolic peel (glycolic acid acts as an exfoliant, sloughing off layers of dead, flaky skin) or microdermabrasion is administered to treat hardened skin. Nails are then bleached (if necessary) and clipped to perfection. In the meantime, touch up polish with a clear topcoat once a week to keep color from fading or buff nails for a glossy finish. Most of all, says Serquinia, "find ways to take care of yourself now. This is the only package you get—don't deny yourself."

*Handle Yourself
with Care*

7 *H*ONOR *Y*OUR *C*ROWN

"Start with what you know and build on what you have."

—Kwame Nkrumah, 1909–1972;
first president of Ghana

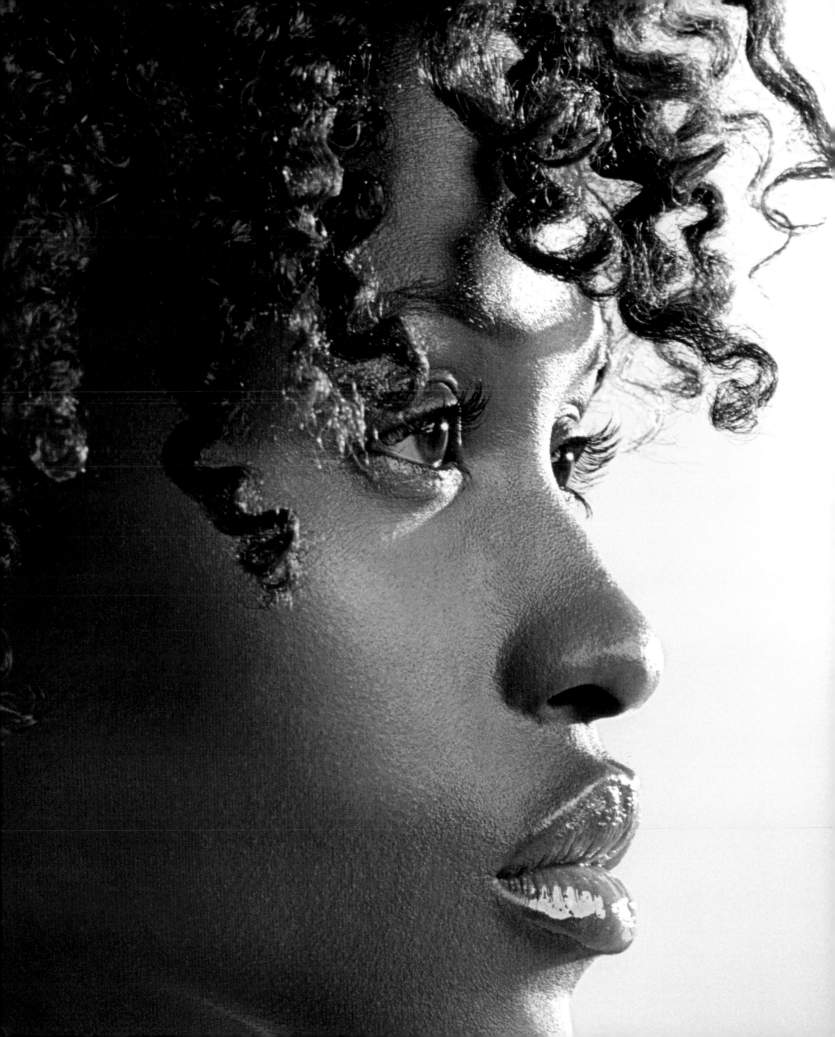

SELF-SEDUCTION

PREVIOUS SPREAD:
Model Aiesha Cain

Growing up in a beauty parlor in the mid-'60s was a pretty heady experience. It was an era when come Saturday, a sister's first priority was getting her hair done to the nines! I would sit and watch them as they strode into my mother's salon right in the heart of Newark, New Jersey, to fulfill their fantasies through the do of their desires. To this day, I clearly remember the distinct odor of bergamot as heated by so many pressing combs and the clicking of curling irons here and there, while sisters shared their confidences about everything from their love life to their beauty. Back then women believed certain stylists had what was known in the community as "growing hands," and naturally everybody wanted to be in their chairs. My mother was one of those gurus from the moment she retired from the showbiz arena. She became known as someone who could turn your hair around, giving you a press that lasted and a head-turning look to go with it. Far from being anyone's magician, what she actually did was start women on a regime, stop them from being too experimental, and get them to commit to it. "Mo," as she was affectionately known by everyone, was also an award-winning colorist who helped many of her swanky customers dream a world, from blond to black cherry and every shade in between! The caveat was that they maintain the health of their hair and visit the salon for professional treatments, which they did, and along with this, most of them kept to their natural hair. My mother was determined that if her reputation was going to be destroyed, she would take care of that herself, as opposed to letting a client who refused to take care of her hair have that privilege. So, needless to say, she was very cautious when it came to the subject of hair straighteners—which were still a real case of trial and error, as manufacturers had yet to turn them into the conditioning relaxers we're familiar with today. So the sisters came and invested their time—having deep conditioners and feeding their spirits with lots of fellowship under hooded dryers—and their hard-earned dollars to go through a transformation process that affirmed how they felt about themselves and polished their crowns.

Later on, a very liberating movement began to take shape within our communities. Sisters (and brothers) were beginning to wear their hair in what was then seen (and secretly feared) by many as a symbolic tool of power—an Afro! Every size, shade, and shape of this style ruled, calling for an array of diverse tools and products to accompany a new mind-set about our distinctive beauty. A proclamation was issued—"Black is beautiful"—and more and more of us joined the movement away from our former aesthetic and embraced our hair in all its natural glory. During the '70s we carried on with our crowns both on the big screen and in the streets. Afros continued to rule, perms expertly took us into new territory, and color made our wildest dreams come true! By the time the '80s rolled around cuts were a mainstay, with wedged bobs and blunt cuts being a tour de force. Curly perms allowed us to spritz, shake, and go live the fast-paced life of our desires. Cornrows were also moving across the scene, with some of the most intricate designs imaginable, giving us a break from the daily styling grind while causing great disturbance in the workplace at the same time. And so the '90s ushered in a hard-won freedom—the ability to embrace a look based on one's individuality and the drive to explore all our options, not conformity. Many of us embraced ultra-short hair to haute extremes—from microcuts and short naturals to bald heads—and I loved us for being so bold. This mental movement continues to give new meaning to the concept of being creative and has yielded some of the most incredible styles, texture choices, and color techniques we've ever known.

Through it all, no matter what the era, our hair has always been both a barometer of style and an indication of how we felt about ourselves. Since the dawn of our existence, our hair has been a self-defined crown. With skilled hands we have crafted and styled our rich, distinctive textures. We used clay from the dust of the earth to color our hair—a befitting backdrop for the art that adorned our faces and the scarification that set off our bodies. It was only during the dark years of slavery that we were not allowed to display our hair, let alone have the time to administer to it in the ways we were accustomed to. Snatched from the cradle of civilization, without our loved ones, our tools, or the ability to embrace our aesthetic, we produced styles that were distinctly different from those we were accustomed to creating. This debilitating experience, which robbed us of our dignity and crushed our spirits, did yield a basic plaiting style, one that we continue to proudly display to this day. With a legacy of such tragedy and adversity, it is without a doubt a true testament that we survived and went on to triumph.

Today, when you think about it, no other group of people on earth has had or continues to have as much controversy over the characteristics of their hair as we have. This unwelcome attention has manifested itself in many ways over the years, but never more powerfully within us as the good-hair-versus-bad-hair syndrome. Back in the day, "good hair" meant hair that was straight, and often long. "Bad hair" was hair that was kinky, woolly, in need of so-called taming, and (according to erroneous theory) unable to grow. But as we began to refute this thinking and appreciate our hair's uniqueness, we began to work what we had so richly been given, without limiting it from within, all of which got us to the liberating freedom that we enjoy today—a freedom that allows us to explore our options with a deliberate passion. In fact, I'm convinced it's our passion for change that continues to inspire manufacturers to create the wide array of product choices enabling us to fully act upon our desires like no other generation of sisters before. Yes, we have emerged, but now it's up to us to maintain this victory by taking only the soundest approach to styling and caring for our hair. Moreover, dare I say, we have to maintain this victory from the inside out. Author Alice Walker told me several years ago that she has a spiritual relationship with her hair. Stroking her locks lovingly as she spoke, she went on to reveal to me that her locks were an extension of herself. At first I marveled at her declaration, but by the end of our time spent together, I realized that Walker appreciates and honors her body; her hair is no exception to that mode of thinking. If you appreciate and honor your hair, you won't do it wrong! You won't allow yourself to slide into a pattern of thinking that allows you to treat your hair as if it is only there for your most disposable desires. Instead, you'll choose your options with discernment and reject those practices that take more than they give. More often than not, those are the ones that put us on the path to damage control anyway. I can say that without any fear of contradiction because I've been there and done that and I know the perils firsthand. In fact, there was a time when I thought I knew more about my hair than my stylist. It was during this know-it-all phase that I convinced her against her will to permanently color and relax my fine, fragile hair. Well a few weeks later, while she was blow-drying my hair it began drifting across the floor! You don't need me to tell you how painful this was— losing my hair in a very public space due to my own stubbornness. Well, I just licked my wounds and followed her advice for recovery, which included intensive conditioning, repeated trims, and a restful style without any tension. Today, we keep it simple. My fine hair is still relaxed, but *temporary* color is used to create the espresso brown hue I favor. Weekly conditioners that revolve around hot oil treatments and protein conditioners as needed, or an oil bath and a cream conditioner for extra hydration, keep my strands strong, supple, and shiny. Scalp treatments that address my specific needs also play a role. These treatments are key due to the environmental and lifestyle concerns that could pose a problem for my hair. For example, my hair takes a beating from perspiration during my workouts, and dry cabin air from lots of plane travel saps my best efforts at times for keeping it hydrated. Like many of us, I use a leave-in conditioner and am careful with the kind as well as the amount of styling aids I use, but nevertheless, none of this is a substitute for professional care and products.

Although my hair loss was only temporary, it all said to me that in order to have and keep healthy hair, I needed to weigh all the options—especially any of a chemical nature—with expert guidance. The first time I visited bio-esthetician and stylist George Buckner of Hair Fashion's East Salon in New York City, my hair was in serious trouble. I had been experiencing dryness and a lot of breakage. Buckner analyzed a strand of my hair under a microscope and told me he could tell each of my most recent relaxer touch-ups, as there were bumps of unevenness throughout the shaft. I immediately confessed that I was in between stylists and had been chemically straightening and caring for my hair at home. I decided right then and there that *I* would stop trying to be a professional stylist and consult one as I had clearly done my hair an injustice.

Any chemical process must take into consideration your hair and its condition, something that requires professional knowledge. Finally, commit to honoring your hair by giving it the TLC it needs. Styling trends come and go, but the care of your hair must remain consistent, and everything else must flow from this basic principle of care first, style second. When we were growing up, our mothers kept this strategy in mind through their self-created principle of rest and display. During the week, most of us wore our hair in braids or soft ponytails. But come Sunday, we got the cleverest creations one can imagine, with curls and twists and all kinds of adornments. This wasn't an everyday occurrence; otherwise our hair would have been taxed from childhood. To me, we need to keep this same principle in mind when we approach the styling of our hair—restful styling and practices during the week and then those that call for the works on special occasions. It stands to reason that too many days of doing whatever it takes to achieve a high-maintenance look—whether constant curling, sleeping in rollers, overuse of holding products, or too frequent chemical touch-ups—will eventually take its toll on hair. Better, then, to be discerning and customize our styling, care, and any chemical treatments with the health of our hair at the forefront, because it's about starting with what we know, and then consciously building upon what we have.

Hair Growth: The Perfect Flow

Looking at the number of pomades and supplements claiming to make hair grow, one would think that miracles were finally available at a price! The reality is, hair grows from within, not without. "Nothing topical has been proven to make hair grow," says noted dermatologist Jeanine B. Downie. And while vitamin supplements do support our bodies, those aimed at making hair grow primarily contain the same ingredients as your high-potency multivitamin, so don't be misled!

As ordered by our Creator, hair starts growing in the womb! Once we're born, it is nourished beneath the scalp and grows a quarter inch to a half inch every month. During your lifetime, it is always engaged in one of three phases: the growth phase (anagen), the rest or dormant stage (catagen), and the shedding phase (telegen), where hair drops off and is replaced by new strands. According to Dallas trichologist Rodney Barnett, "if you are healthy, eighty-five percent of your hair should be in the growing cycle at all times." This perfect flow is sustained by good health, diet, and lifestyle. This is where we come in, and how well we manage our temples plays a key role in our hair and its growth from within. Experts tell us that hair is first nourished internally through nutrients in our blood. Therefore, a healthy diet is inextricably bound to healthy hair. Another reason why consulting a nutritionist is so important is that it's more than helpful to have the kind of information that will guide you to a *balanced* diet that supplies all of your needs, which change periodically throughout your lifetime.

Curl Interrupted!

Our hair, despite its being the most fragile hair on earth, spirals upward on a determined growth cycle, resulting in an array of the most beautiful textures, on course. There have been many times, however, when I've heard sisters say, "My hair won't grow." Unless impacted by stress, extreme dieting, illness, medications, or heat and chemical burns that have permanently damaged hair follicles, nothing interrupts that flow. There are many external factors that can prevent you from retaining your growth, all of which are within your control, but the work your body does from within proceeds on course unless otherwise jolted by very serious circumstances. "Often our hair is breaking at the same rate of growth, so we never see the length," offers Downie. There are also things that can impact hair loss or thinning, such as heredity, menopause, chemotherapy, chronic stress, weight-loss programs, prescribed medications, or an undetected hormonal imbalance. Stress is a common issue for us today. "When a person is under stress, the body's adrenal system is affected. Adrenaline, which is a hormone, prepares the body for 'flight, fright, or fight' when under stress and creates a temporary imbalance internally," says Barnett. This has an impact on your entire system (digestive, circulatory, nervous, etc.), causing it to not operate at an optimal level. It's important to note that when there is an imbalance going on, the body won't compromise the major organs—rather, "it will sacrifice the extras, like skin, hair and nails," he adds. According to Downie, systemic diseases or health conditions can also disrupt the system and possibly affect the hair. "After major surgery, systems have to repair themselves, and hair could certainly be affected," she says. So anything that impacts our internal systems can have a direct impact on hair's growth cycle.

On the other hand, when it comes to hair loss or even thinning, take action. Don't suffer in silence; rather, empower yourself by getting the necessary facts. Ask your doctor if any of the medications you are taking could have possibly affected the condition of your hair, and if so, whether there are alternatives. For loss or thinning that may be a result of other conditions indicated, enlist the help of a dermatologist or a trichologist (a specialist in hair and scalp disorders). You might also call on the help of a naturopathic doctor or a herbalist for a strategy. And don't rule out tending your inner beauty during such an emotional experience. Be encouraged to seek the affirming guidance you need from within through therapy. Finally, stay in partnership with your hair care professional, who can offer styling alternatives or even work with you to create a savvy wig to allow you to keep stepping in style while on the rebound!

Mane Stays

"Everyone's hair grows approximately six inches a year. To keep those inches you need to take care of them with a good conditioning regimen," says veteran stylist Olive Benson, owner of Olive's Beauty Salon in Boston, Massachusetts. Unfortunately, Benson notes, today's fast-paced lifestyles and attitudes about hair care mean that conditioning is something that often gets put on the back burner. "Everyone who comes into the salon wants low-maintenance hair. Rarely is this possible for Black women unless their hair is extremely short," she adds. Even if for no other reason than the fact that you want to push the envelope when it comes to style, you need to make conditioning a priority. Says hairstylist Oscar James, who keeps the look of many A-list celebrities and models, "It's really about pampering—so condition, condition, condition." For hair that's as dry and delicate as ours due to its natural curl pattern, moisture is essential. Weekly treatments that hydrate and/or strengthen and daily leave-in conditioners should play a role in our regimens without fail. From there, it's about the prescribed care of a knowledgeable stylist to address your unique needs, and a real commitment to yourself to tend your hair as directed. "There just isn't any miracle," concludes stylist extraordinaire André Walker, who keeps Oprah Winfrey's hair lush and lovely. "You can't have beautiful and healthy hair if you don't take the time to do what it takes. It's like working out—you've got to do it—so you've got to find a way to put it in your schedule."

Experts urge us to not let trends dictate so much that we forgo health for style. "Healthy hair *is* stylish," says James. Therefore, you need to make discerning choices when it comes to styling practices, as this is an area that can easily prevent growth retention through breakage as well as unhealthy, lackluster locks. To that end, bridging the gap between the hair that we possess and the hair we desire comes about first from within. "I think we need to be able to come to terms with what we have and knowing what it can do and how we can make the best of it," Walker points out. Just about every move you make, from sleeping on cotton pillowcases (drying) to combing, brushing, and even shampooing incorrectly, has an impact on your hair. Even water quality plays a role. Then there are those practices that really compromise hair's health, such as frequent use of heated appliances, tight braiding and other tension-driven styles, and styling aids that offer "super hold." "Hair needs to rest from heat, excessive styling, extremes," says Barnett, all of which can weaken it and lead to breakage.

These and other truths call for us to take a healthy approach to how we treat our hair. Seeking out the best professional care and then working in partnership with that stylist is the first step on the road to preserving your hair. Simply put, you need to see your stylist for all chemical services as well as to interpret the condition of your hair and what it can and cannot take. Most celebrities and women in the know have that certain someone that they entrust their hair to. They don't move around from stylist to stylist, trying new things as they go. "Oprah knows I know her hair and she listens to me and does what it takes. So I know if Oprah's hair falls out, it's either me or her—somebody has done something wrong!" Walker points out. This kind of relationship calls for you to be informed by knowing exactly what is being used on your hair and why, and it also calls for you to use only the most nurturing products that impart moisture and condition your hair, as opposed to taking from it with drying agents and other elements that may not be suitable for it.

Loving Care

There's no secret when it comes to what will keep hair strong, supple, and healthy. It requires a loving care regimen based on expert technique and appropriate products. Here's your checklist:

SHAMPOO Because our needs can and do change, choosing the proper shampoo is essential. "Do look for those rich in moisture, especially if you have relaxed hair, so you cleanse without stripping the hair," says stylist Oscar James. Look to such humectants as wheat amino acids or silk amino acids. Select only those that address your specific needs. For example, if you work out multiple times a week, choose a shampoo that's safe for frequent use, to prevent drying your hair out. If you wear braids, be sure to choose a shampoo that won't leave a damaging residue between them—a gel formula, as opposed to a creamy one. If you have dandruff and have relaxed hair, make sure to use a shampoo that checks it without the high sudsing usually associated with many shampoos of this type, as it will strip much-needed oils from your hair. In general, look to those that gently cleanse, leaving a soft slip to your hair as opposed to a squeaky clean finish, which will cause you an immense amount of tangling. Above all, consult your stylist about which brands and types are best for you.

COMING CLEAN

A host of shampoo types exist to safely cleanse your hair without stripping it of its natural oils. Here is a mini review of those that may be appropriate for you depending on your needs and the condition of your hair and scalp:

- **Protein: cleanses buildup, slight strengthening benefits**

- **Conditioning/moisturizing: cleanse, coat, and protect the hair**

- **Clarifying: cleanses product buildup from styling aids**

- **Dandruff: checks flaky scalps**

- **Color-treated: deposits pigment and protects color from fading during the cleansing process**

CONDITIONER By and large, the characteristics of our hair mean you want to impart moisture at every opportunity, from a daily leave-in conditioner to making time for those that penetrate through the addition of heat. "If breakage is a problem, a protein conditioner to strengthen hair" is in order, according to James, who adds, "Now there are some that won't leave the hair hard," a real concern in the past. You can also try this tip at home from stylist Barry Fletcher of Maryland's Avant Garde Hair Gallery, in Seat Pleasant: "Take an egg and add it to your moisturizing conditioner to get the benefit of raw protein." Hot oil treatments are also a real boon for dry hair. Recognizing that conditioning is so paramount, today many stylists will coat previously relaxed hair with a conditioner to prevent overprocessing before giving their clients a relaxer touch-up. Most importantly, be sure to use a conditioner every time you wash your hair, because some natural oils are removed during the cleansing phase, and your hair needs to be replenished.

SCALP CARE Back in the day, our mothers used to "grease" our scalps. They meant well, but oftentimes the petroleum-based pomades they used were too heavy. However, today there are a host of lightweight products designed specifically to care for the scalp. Many revitalize and cancel dryness and itchiness without a greasy buildup. Just be sure to avoid those that contain such scalp-clogging ingredients as glycerin, beeswax, and again, petroleum. On the professional end, many incorporate essential oils with molecules small enough to penetrate the scalp and stimulate circulation. To this end, routine massages to stimulate the scalp and lift dead cells are something that you can easily do a few times a week as well. "Rubber scalp brushes (sold at beauty supply stores) that don't scratch the scalp are also good," adds Annu Prestonia of the Khamit Kinks Salon, in New York City, which specializes in the care and styling of natural hair. Any scalp condition, such as bumps that may develop as a result of tight braiding, should be seen by a dermatologist or a trichologist, as this signals an infection and could lead to permanent hair loss. How so? Each time hair follicles are infected, they heal with a bit of scar tissue. Over time, if this happens again and again, the follicles close up for good.

CUTTING Incumbent with the stress of styling is a fair degree of wear and tear to our hair, particularly the ends. If you think about it, the ends of your hair represent the most aged portion—in other words, the part that has endured the most aggression. Keeping them from stressing the rest of your hair is key. "Just like a pair of jeans without a hem, the ends will fray and split and work their way up the strands," says stylist Marvin A. Carrington of New York City's Jelani Hair Salon. To prevent this from happening and ultimately destroying your hair, have ends trimmed every four to six weeks. Be sure to buffer this section of your hair with a little extra conditioner, especially when using heat appliances. And always use end papers when roller-setting. Aside from the health of your ends, we know that a cut is a key styling essential that shaves time off of our morning regimens and makes the occurrence of "bad hair days" something we don't even have to think about. "A haircut is the foundation of a hairstyle, so it's important to go *every* month to six weeks and get it done," says Walker.

In truth, these are nothing if not the modern times we dreamed of. There are more styling aids available than ever to shape, control, and polish our hair to perfection. However, everything out there isn't for the taking. And even among those products that are suitable there's room for tweaking. Personally, I think your choice of stylers should be directed by your hair care professional. On this end of the spectrum you should be using what he or she uses to finish your look, or selecting the retail items your stylist advises. It's also important to make sure that the aids you use have synergy. On any given day we sisters can have three or four styling aids in our hair (leave-in conditioner, holding product, sheen spray, etc.). Therefore it's important that they all work together without causing any adverse effect on your hair, or at the very least won't give your hair a filmy finish. Sometimes there's a need to add additional moisture, especially when utilizing holding products. On a personal note, I find this to be the case and therefore add a light liquid oil to a straightening balm to smooth and hydrate my hair at the same time. The use of the straightening balm, by the way, allows for a sleek, straight finish without undue tension or the use of heat more than once a week to get me there. So having a coterie of styling aids that you can trust is more than important. Here are two modern-day survival checklists, one for relaxed hair and one for natural hair, to guide you in your choices:

RELAXED HAIR

- Light pomade—to promote health, lock in moisture, buff against heat, add shine, and help ends stay in place

- Liquid oil—to protect, add lubrication, hold moisture, smooth, add shine

- Leave-in conditioner—to treat, impart moisturizers, and buff hair from root to ends during heat styling

- Light holding spritz—preferably alcohol-free; allows for a flexible hold and light control overall

- Sheen spray—to add glossy shine overall without buildup

- Anti-frizz agent—to prevent frizz and keep hair smooth; great for use around the hairline

- Alcohol-free styling gel—to impart control and smooth hair as needed; great for stray edges

- Setting lotion—for wraps and smooth roller sets

- Conditioning mousse—to create fullness, give a slight hold

- Pomade—opt for a botanically based cream pomade to reduce buildup, promote health, lubricate, lock in moisture, and repel frizzing; avoid those that are heavy or waxy in order to prevent buildup and attraction of dust and pollution

- Shea butter—to hydrate, treat, protect

- Liquid oil—a natural oil, such as sweet almond, jojoba, or sesame, that can be customized with essential oils for added benefits; to condition, lubricate, hold moisture, impart shine

- Leave-in conditioner—to treat, lubricate, impart moisturizers, add shine

- Gel—to smooth hairline and create hold: twists, knots, and other set styles

- Sheen spray—to add glossy shine overall without buildup

- Scalp aid—to hydrate and prevent itching

Pro Tips!

What does it take in addition to a great care regimen to have and maintain the hair of your desires? Professional know-how. Here, the experts give us the best-ever beauty advice on some of our most popular style moves.

BLOW-DRYING

"Always use a professional-grade dryer—
from 1,200 to 1,500 watts, to get enough heat
to straighten hair—and a good comb attachment."
MARVIN A. CARRINGTON, JELANI SALON, NEW YORK CITY

"Incorporating the right products from the beginning—from shampoo to conditioner—is essential. For great results, blow-dry hair in the direction of the style you desire and when seventy-five percent dry add a dab of oil throughout. And if you get most of the water out of the hair before using the comb attachment you'll get a silkier, softer finish."
BARRY FLETCHER, AVANT GARDE HAIR GALLERY,
SEAT PLEASANT, MARYLAND

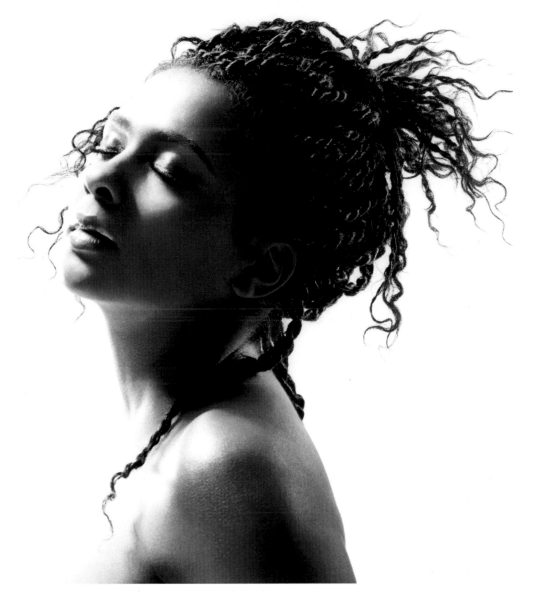

"Before drying, always use a styling agent to protect the hair, and always use a comb attachment. You can really damage the hair using a brush if you don't know what you're doing."

DIANA NURSE, EXPECTATIONS AND INNOVATIONS SALON, NEW YORK CITY

"The secret is what you put in before—use a blow-drying cream so your hair will stay straight longer. And always towel-dry the hair first; never blow-dry dripping-wet hair!"

CELEBRITY STYLIST OSCAR JAMES

"Blow-drying is step one of your hairstyle—it is the foundation!"

CELEBRITY STYLIST ANDRÉ WALKER

Model Tammy Ford

There are so many textures available to us today when it comes to choosing hair for extension styling. Making the right choice, whether you're looking for a fresh, scissored pixie, a sassy, razor-cut bob, or long, sensuous layers, hinges on a variety of considerations, from your lifestyle and how much time you have to devote to maintenance, to why you've chosen extension styling, whether it be to achieve a certain look, give hair a rest from chemicals, or recover from and camouflage damage. To simplify your decision and select that which is in your best interest, it's best to have a professional consultation with a qualified expert who can guide you both to a suitable style as well as the type of hair that should be used. However, even if you don't choose to go this route, it's best to approach your choices like a professional. In general, when it comes to the most natural-looking weaves and braided do's, celebrity stylist Ellin LaVar, who's behind such best-tressed celebs as Missy Elliott, Naomi Campbell, and Whitney Houston, urges sisters first and foremost to make sure that the look you choose is realistic for you. As part of her consultation, LaVar weighs such details as your natural hairline, the shape of your head, the length of your hair, what style you're choosing, and the thickness of your natural hair, as well as your profession and lifestyle. "Then we ascertain what look the client is trying to present most of the time and give them something versatile that allows them to wear a style that's appropriate for work, but permits them to go funky on the weekend," says LaVar.

Equally important is the care and condition of your own hair and scalp. Whatever style you choose to wear, it is of the utmost importance that you have access to your scalp and that the process doesn't cause trauma to it or to your natural hair. LaVar cites such important techniques as nourishing the scalp with a conditioner, weekly shampooing, and conditioning overall, with particular care to your natural hair wherever it is exposed. You should also choose those products that will keep your look healthy and lustrous. LaVar recommends "moisturizing shampoos, shampoos for color-treated hair to keep it from being dry and brittle, leave-in conditioners, and moisturizing creams instead of oils for daily maintenance, as oils just sit on top of the hair," she explains. For certain you want to avoid styling aids with alcohol, as they will cause dryness and dull the hair, making it look totally fake—not cute! To keep your look salon-fresh and prevent matting, be sure to wrap your hair at night with a silky scarf or a satin bonnet, or if you wear braids, a stocking cap to keep it in place and frizz-free. Remember your nighttime objective is to continue to pamper your hair, so it's important to avoid the culprits of cotton—as in scarves and pillowcases—which dry hair out and cause friction if your natural hair is exposed and unprotected, which weakens and causes breakage.

When selecting hair for a weave, what's key to a natural finish is choosing a texture that complements your own if you intend to incorporate your natural hair as part of the look you desire. Human hair is usually best, as it places the least amount of stress on your own hair and offers you a greater range of style, texture, and color options. Human hair extensions can be heat-styled, roller set, colored, and cut to move like your own hair. Many celebrities and models work their style and color options to the hilt through this very process, saving their own hair from the stress of double-processing and lots of heat. If you're a sister who likes to switch up often, for example from long to short, straight to textured, or from brunette to blond, human hair extensions can offer you the experience minus the long-term commitment, let alone the avoidance of stressing your own hair. On the other hand, I've seen many a stylist work some of the finest synthetic textures technology has made possible, yielding the most fabulous 'fros and other au naturel looks that would take your breath away! So it's really a question of weighing your options, evaluating your lifestyle and what's required to maintain the look you have in mind, as well as placing yourself in the hands of an expert stylist with a great resource for quality extensions and style know-how. As for braids, both human and synthetic hair offer you a wide range of options. In this case, there are pros and cons to both. Some styles just translate better using synthetic hair as opposed to human, as it stays neater longer and is sturdier. However, according to LaVar, synthetic hair is rougher on our natural hair because it tends to both cut the hair and dry it out. Human hair extensions, which tend to be softer, more compatible with your own hair, and offer you greater versatility, require more maintenance. "Human hair expands when washed, so it doesn't stay as neat looking as synthetic hair without tying it down and using gels to maintain it," notes LaVar.

Regardless of the style and texture you choose, experts say it's critical that we protect the health of our own hair by not weighing it down with too much added hair, which weakens strands and leads to breakage, or worse yet, permanent hair loss, and by choosing a method of application that again, doesn't traumatize your scalp in the process. And along these lines, know that it's important that you follow your salon professional's advice regarding touch-ups and care, especially that of trimming of the ends of your hair, especially if it's natural, to prevent frizzies. In general, it's best to have your weave tightened every six to eight weeks and to shampoo and condition hair weekly, making sure to comb the hair out from the ends to the base and always dry it thoroughly using a hooded dryer before you begin any styling methods, with the exception of a roller-set. Blow-drying (which allows you to achieve faster, sleeker results) or the use of a diffuser (which will dry curly textures leaving them intact in no time) doesn't effectively dry the base of your weave, and in the case of blow-drying, places additional stress on both the extensions and your own hair. For braided do's, providing you have a style that allows you to shampoo and condition your hair weekly—unlike Goddess Braids, for example—it's important to follow your stylist's advice for the particular look you are wearing. Many stylists will recommend that you minimize the amount of time you leave synthetic extensions in due to the fact that it zaps moisture from the hair, advising removal after a four- to six-week period, followed by deep conditioning of your natural hair. In general, you are advised to have regular touch-ups, whether you wear human hair or synthetic extensions and to never go longer than two months without doing so, as you risk damaging your own hair.

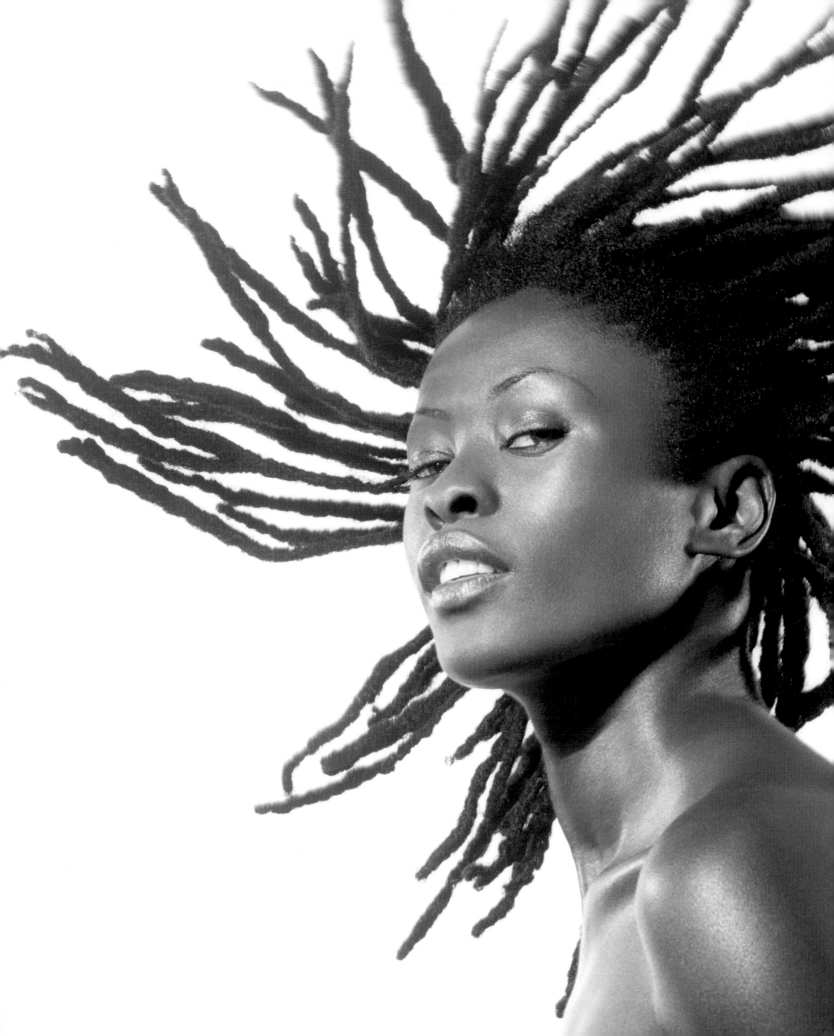

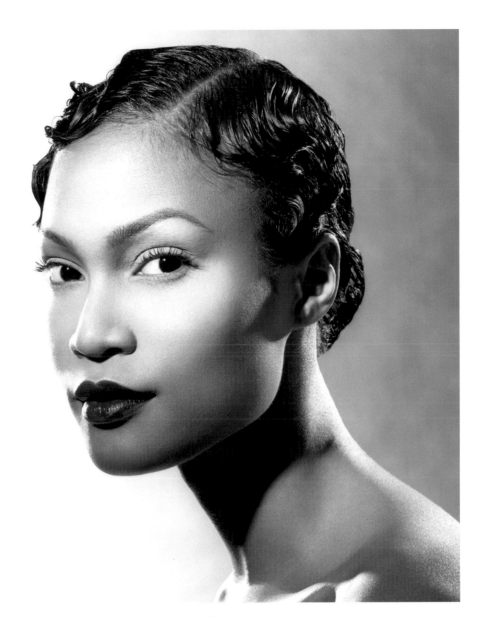

PRESSING

"There are over eighteen different textures
of curly hair, and most of us need the stove method for a truly straight finish,
which is why this should be done by a professional."

MARVIN A. CARRINGTON

"Technique is more important than product—
it's elbow grease and the back of the iron that
ensure sleekness."

**KEITH CAMPBELL, C.O.I. STUDIO,
BROOKLYN, NEW YORK**

OPPOSITE:

Model Laurence Basse

ABOVE:

Model Crystal Wong

CURLING/IRONING

"Wet-setting before curling with an iron
will give curls more memory, making them
last longer."

BARRY FLETCHER

"You have to be careful how hot the
iron is, which is why I like thermostatically
controlled irons."

CELEBRITY STYLIST DERRICK SCURRY

"Always use an iron on clean hair *only*."

DIANA NURSE

ROLLER-SETTING

"Always set trimmed ends!"

BARRY FLETCHER

"At all times use a setting lotion to prevent frizzies, and make
sure hair is completely dry before you release rods or rollers."

DERRICK SCURRY

"Use plastic rollers—gives a smoother set than mesh rollers."

ANNU PRESTONIA, KHAMIT KINKS SALON, NEW YORK CITY

"Always good for fullness! Most of the looks you get with a curling iron
you can get with setting. In this way the more time you spend
the better for your hair."

OSCAR JAMES

"A paddle brush is great for loosening tight curls without
canceling out body."

DARYLE BENNETT, NEW YORK CITY

WRAPPING

"Take your time and use a fine-toothed comb to avoid bumps and unevenness to
your finished look. Always use a wrap lotion to help the hair remember the shape."

MARVIN A. CARRINGTON

"Make sure hair is thoroughly dry before you disturb a wrap."

DIANA NURSE

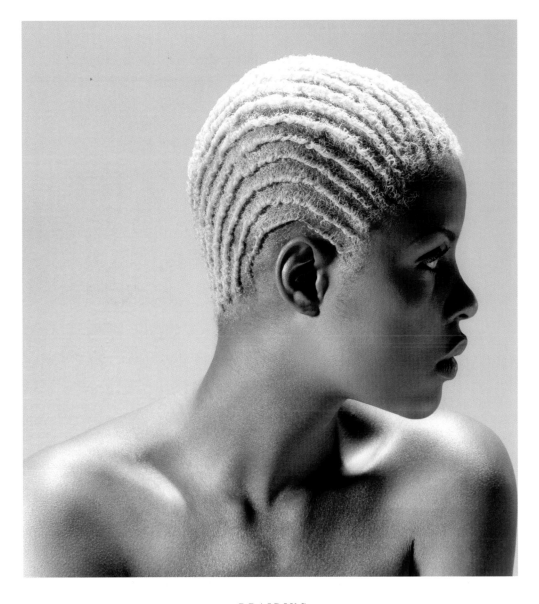

BRAIDING

"Don't sacrifice health for style! Using an excessive amount of extensions
on a small amount of natural hair will create atrophy, breakage and lead
to traction alopecia!"

DIANE BAILEY, TENDRILS SALON FOR NATURAL HAIR AND WELLNESS,BROOKLYN, NEW YORK

"Make sure to remove braids and shampoo as well as deep-condition
your hair every four to six weeks for the *optimum* health of your hair."

BARRY FLETCHER

"Tight braiding techniques lead to traction alopecia, especially at the hairline.
I'd rather see fuzzies than lost hair!"

**DR. JEANINE B. DOWNIE, IMAGE CENTER
FOR DERMATOLOGY, MONTCLAIR, NEW JERSEY**

BRAID REMOVAL

"Remove braids gently without tugging, from the ends to the roots, and always use a product designed for this purpose to prevent breakage and give hair much-needed slip to ease the process."

**DEBRA HARE-BEY, RED CREATIVE SALON,
BROOKLYN, NEW YORK**

"Thoroughly comb out each section to prevent fusing or matting of the hair when you shampoo."

DIANE BAILEY

BONDING

"No way! It's cute for a quick fix, but it's certainly something you don't want to live in. Braided extensions or weaving is healthier for the hair."

OSCAR JAMES

"Glue does not belong on the scalp—it can cause chemically induced scarring alopecia."

DR. JEANINE B. DOWNIE

TOOL TIME

Keeping your tools in the manner your salon professional does not only plays a role in the look of your hair but is a healthy must. Here's how:

- **Clean your combs and brushes once a week with the disinfectant that barbers use—Barbicide.**

- **Replace combs and brushes yearly.**

- **Immediately discard combs with broken or missing teeth.**

- **Cleanse curling irons by first heating them, then unplug and apply a relaxer or an oven cleaner to thoroughly remove all buildup. "Buildup affects the smoothness of your curl," adds Nurse.**

- **Clean rollers once a month in a basin of soap and water with a drop of bleach to kill germs.**

- **Wipe blow-dryers down weekly and wash attachments with soap and water.**

Altered State: Making the Transition from Relaxed to Natural Hair

Because our hair is naturally fragile, any process that alters its already delicate state is one that should be considered thoroughly and handled with the utmost care. Today, as more and more of us turn inward and become more in tune with ourselves, many are making the transition from chemically processed hair back to our hair in its natural state. Making this transition can be a traumatic move if not done with knowledge, care, and restful styles that are long on looks and short on manipulation. To successfully accomplish this while retaining your growth requires a game plan that coddles hair, particularly where the two textures meet, and allows you to keep your style quotient intact during the process.

STRATEGIZE The road back to natural requires care every step of the way. To begin, it's best to determine if yours will be one that's a gradual process or if you'll desire to liberate yourself right from the start with an ultra-savvy short cut! I've seen many sisters take this approach and discover a side of themselves they never knew existed. They are moving through life now with what they deem as the ultimate freedom! On the other hand, many have discovered alternative styling techniques that ease them through this transition without damage and in great style, such as:

- Two-strand twists

- Coils

- Bantu knots

- Straw or rod sets

- Braids

- Faux or true locks

- Weaves

Those who decide to retain their length without putting a stationary style in place have to be the most cautious and aim for looks that can be fingered into shape with as little stress as possible at the point where new growth and relaxed hair meet. Begin by placing the care and styling of your hair in the hands of a professional stylist and select a look that you can master from week to week. In this case a rod set is a good alternative, as it will camouflage the area where the textures meet and allow you to finger-comb your hair into place, lessening your chances of breakage. "As you hair is growing out it's especially important to be moisture-conscious," says stylist Barry Fletcher, since dryness can lead to breakage. Regular trims are also important to the health and look of the hair. Natural-hair wonder Derrick Scurry reminds us that, due to texture variables, "hair in transition cannot be *perfect* every day" in the sense that every hair is in place, which is why many sisters select a stationary style such as those listed above. Most of all, the transition phase represents a time to coddle your hair—with deep-conditioning treatments, protecting it with a silky scarf at night, and keeping it lubricated during the day—and to get acquainted with your natural texture as it emerges. This is also a time to invest in a change of hair tools, beginning with a wide-tooth comb and perhaps a small toothbrush for minimal smoothing of the hairline, especially in the nape area, as well as a change of products to those that are alcohol-free and address both textures of your hair.

The Cool in Hue

I think hair color is one of the biggest cosmetic moves we make, as this is where we're most experimental. We use hair color to warm, highlight, punctuate, switch up, color (*not* cover) gray, and add a touch of drama, just because we've got the panache to do so! From celebrity sisters such as Janet Jackson, Faith Evans, and Beyoncé Knowles to women in the know, we rock color and technique with a passion that's more than visionary. As long as we go to great lengths to deliver such style, we must also work the necessary maintenance to keep our locks in prime condition. It pays, then, to weigh your options wisely and negotiate around such realities as time, upkeep, and the condition of your hair. Here's a point list to keeping your mane brilliant and healthy:

- Work out your options with a professional colorist, who will help you determine your best move according to lifestyle habits (for example, are you a swimmer, or do you exercise frequently?), the cost of the process to your hair as well as your wallet, and how often you're able to visit the salon for touch-ups.

- As any chemical process will cause further dryness, weekly hydrating treatments and leave-in conditioners are a must.

- Protein conditioners to fortify your hair should also be a part of your care regime.

- Maintenance products should all be geared for color-treated hair— these condition, deposit color, and/or protect color from fading.

- If you have permanent color, keep heat styling to a minimum.

COLORFUL CUES

Your glossary at a glance:

Bleach: permanently removes natural pigment; used to highlight, lift color; taxes hair the most

Semi-permanent color: deposits color; lasts six to eight weeks; gentler than permanent color, but still constitutes a double process when applied to relaxed hair

Demi-permanent color: penetrates the hair shaft, doesn't lift, imparts some color; great for color correcting in the hands of a professional; lasts six to eight weeks

Permanent color: incorporates peroxide to create a permanent change; can lift existing color and impart a new one

Conditioning color: imparts conditioning properties onto the hair and coats it during the color process; lasts four to six weeks; safe for relaxed hair

Rinse: does not penetrate, only coats the strands of the hair; enriches existing color; lasts approximately three to four shampoos; safe for relaxed hair

■ Locks can take much longer to absorb color than virgin hair at the roots and often call for additional product. Therefore it's best to have locks colored by a professional, at least initially. A pro will also take into account the age of your locks and be able to determine how often to color them to prevent breakage.

■ To enhance and brighten gray, as well as neutralize any yellow tones, try semi-permanent color in lighter hues.

AT HOME

■ Select at-home products with great care and always patch-test the product on your skin to determine any sensitivities and on a few strands of hair to see if you favor the results.

■ Follow instructions to the letter!

■ Never apply color if scalp is irritated.

■ Deep-condition hair in the weeks leading up to color application and routinely thereafter.

■ Always apply color to clean hair, making sure to cover hair thoroughly from roots to ends for an even tone.

■ If hair is damaged or breaking, see a professional for salon-level conditioning and advice as to when coloring your hair will be appropriate.

■ Wait at least two weeks between relaxer application and coloring.

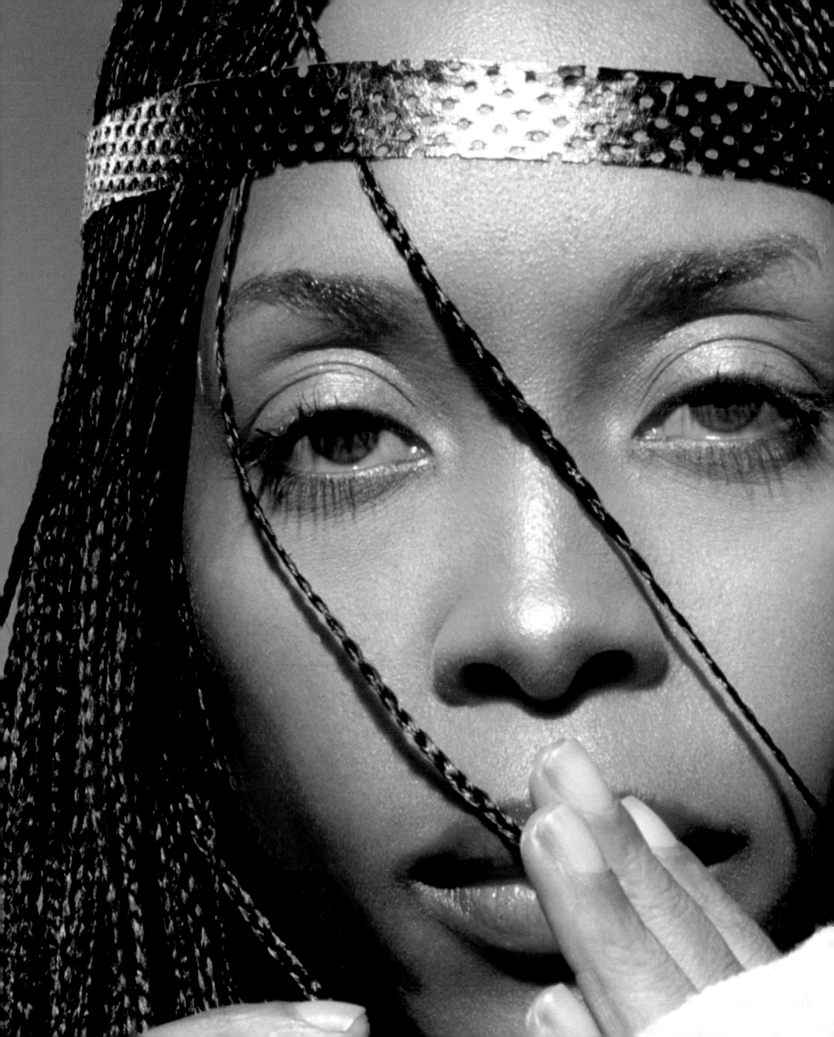

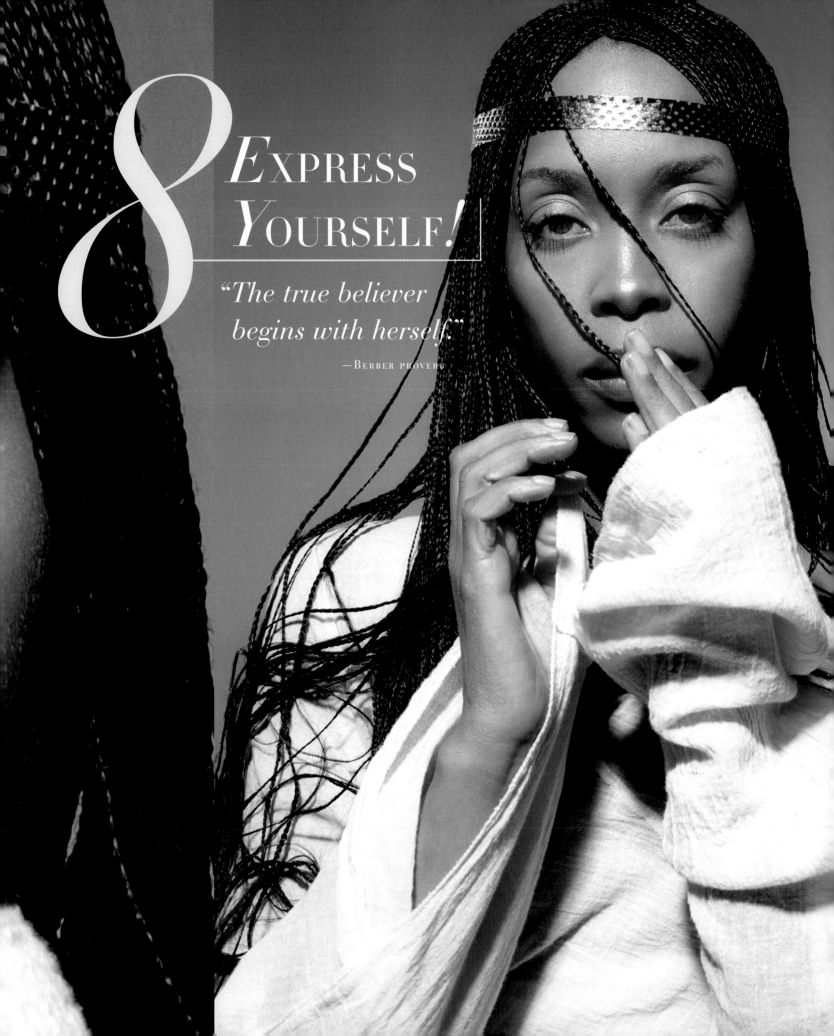

8 Express Yourself!

"The true believer begins with herself."

—Berber proverb

There's nothing more captivating than a woman who knows and understands herself. If style had a definition that you could put your spiritual arms around, to me this would be it. Translating this truth into the tangible when it comes to beauty isn't as mysterious or complicated as you might think. All you need, aside from the confidence to be yourself, is a framework and the ability to have fun exploring yourself within it.

When you are confident, you're more definitive about your choices. You know what works for you and what doesn't. For example, when Sade, one of the savviest music mavens going, stepped off the scene several years ago, she'd made a lasting impression—one that had us loving the easy elegance of pulled-back hair combined with a sassy pair of hoops and red lips. When she returned, I was totally amused, for Sade had simply done a double take on Sade. No image overhaul for her, or any surgical styling (a real stopover for some)—nothing, in fact, to change the woman *she* was comfortable with. Her look had only undergone a subtle but deliberate tweaking to jump it to the present, but without losing that effortless chic she was known for. To me, this represents the anatomy of an attitude, and a woman who knows and understands herself so well that she can work a signature look without it ever becoming dated!

Believe it or not, the same theory holds true for those sisters who possess the creativity to be a chameleon—you know, the ones whose style defies description and always keeps you guessing. These are the sisters who take the concept of "mixing it up" to a higher level. One week their look might be all about Afroesque twists, and just as you get used to that, they turn up with a cropped Caesar! Because they've simply moved on to another space and time on the path to self-discovery, and twists no longer satisfy their souls.

And then there are those who intuitively identify a trademark and work it with gusto. They understand that aside from their overall beauty, there's a certain something that the Creator uniquely placed in their possession, an attribute unequaled in all the earth! And so they can't help but accentuate it to the nth degree.

Truth is, style translates in many ways. For me, it's long been about working a signature look. Like many of us, I'm a working girl and a wife and mother to boot, trying to keep several balls in the air at one time and prevent them from getting away from me. I know just what works with my multitasking lifestyle—a look that's bent on keeping things simple and easy. It occurred to me a long time ago that following each and every trend just wouldn't merge with the pace I need to keep. So I found a framework in which I could fine-tune a look, have a bit of fun, and not compromise my momentum in the process. And mind you, wherever I am in the world, I can turn it out on a dime and not have to think about it anymore! That's not to say I'm in support of a cookie-cutter look. As Iman, who's undoubtedly a chameleon, will quickly tell you, it's not about "staying in some era that you can't get out of." I think getting stuck in a rut is the exact opposite of enjoying one's beauty. Rather, I'm saying the principle of working a signature look is all about finesse. So though I continue to wear my hair in a sleek, no-maintenance style, I now pull it back into a tight little chignon, as opposed to the large bun that used to sit atop my head in the early '90s. And even this look continues to be tweaked, in that the knot changes shape and size, as does the parting of the hair and the makeup and everything else that goes with it, so it all clicks fresh and modern but still says *me*.

Take Creative License

I'm convinced Erykah Badu has got style in her genes. Without question, the three-time Grammy winner is a chameleon who takes the idea of being inventive to another level as well as someone who knows how to work a trademark. "I'm an artist, and so I love to create something on myself, and when I come up with some beautiful creative thing that I feel is very original, I feel really good," says the singer, whose debut forever changed the music scene with her distinct fusion of jazz, R&B, and hip-hop influences. Badu, who's gone from tall majestic head wraps to sigh for—which she still wears and concedes are her trademark—to the bold move of a shaved head, says aside from the fact that beauty is all about creativity

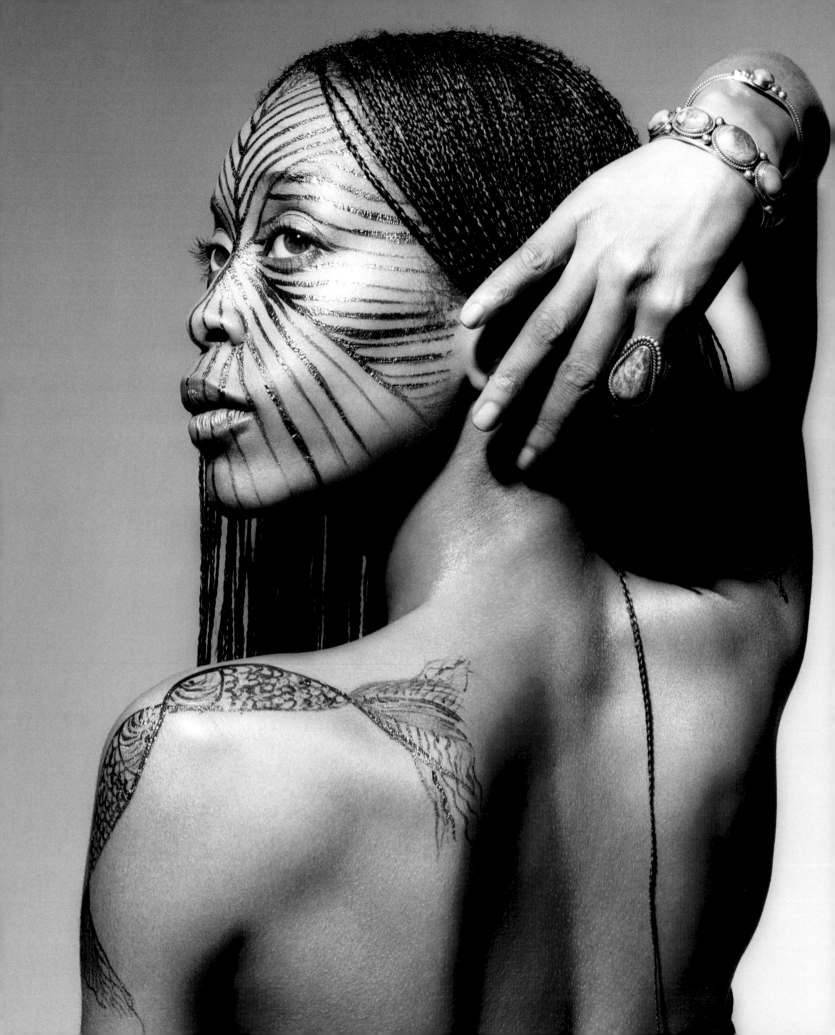

to her, there's also another philosophy behind the changes. "I try not to put myself into a penitentiary psychology, where I'm locked into one thing that people expect from me. It hinders your growth, and you can't grow in God's speed," she adds. In the end, Badu concludes that you're only as free as you think you are. It is this belief that allows her to take creative license and explore waist-length braids, henna designs, and artistic body painting, such as you see here. No doubt as easily as she shaves her head, Badu will continue to shrug off anything expected. Perhaps even by the time you see these images, she'll be on to the next wave.

Truly, there is no formula for taking creative license when it comes to your beauty—it's an intuitive thing. However, I find that women who do so successfully have these things in common:

- Determine their own style

- Are involved in constant self-renewal

- Remain in sync with their entire self

- Are bent on having fun

- Live without hesitation

- Listen within

Eye It!

Identifying and accentuating a beauty trademark is another way to explore your beauty and have a whole lot of fun in the process. For the sister who's been billed as a "director's dream," actress and singer Vanessa Williams, it's always been those compelling eyes that gained her many compliments from the brothers while growing up and now hold the world captive from the theater to the big screen. Williams, who inherited her distinctive blue-gray eyes from her paternal grandfather, says she grew up knowing it was her eyes and today loves casting them in a dramatic light when playing with makeup. "I usually go for a smoky look, using a dark charcoal gray liner with a silver tinge on the lid as well as underneath my lower lashes and then pencil inside the lower lid with a deep black." This immediately creates contrast with her pale eyes and offers a beguiling impact in very little time.

There are many ways to eye your options, no matter what their color, from playing with textures like matte and cream finishes or adding touches of shine and shimmer to working a shade palette you love. Most of all, it's about preserving their beauty. Here's what you need to know:

Erykah Badu

- Have yearly exams.

- Avoid repeated use of eyedrops to check redness, as these contain chemicals that temporarily tighten blood vessels. Select those that are labeled "artificial tears" and preservative-free.

- Keep fragile skin around the eyes hydrated and smooth with products designed specifically for this purpose. Look for those with such moisture-binding ingredients as sodium hyaluronate or hyaluronic acid and cholesterol, linoleic acid or ceramides.

- For puffiness, which can be caused by several factors, including lack of sleep, salt intake, allergies, alcohol consumption, dehydration, and more, try cold cucumber slices, tea bags, or an eye gel or balm containing an anti-inflammatory ingredient such as green tea or herbal extracts such as chamomile, comfrey, or horsetail. Sleep with your head slightly elevated so fluids won't settle in this area.

- To address fine lines, a result of the aging process and too much sun, select technology-driven creams that plump the skin and encourage the production of collagen with ingredients such as glycolic acid, vitamin A, and proteins.

- To improve upon dark circles, which can be a result of insufficient sleep or indicate a circulatory concern, try eye products containing kojic acid, vitamin E derivatives, and anti-inflammatories, along with cream concealers and pressed powder. If they persist, consult your physician.

- Discard makeup as follows: mascara, every three months; eye shadow and pencils, every three to six months.

- Protect skin around the eyes with UV-filtering sunglasses

Serve Lip Appeal

Model Wyinnetka Aaron says she's known for a while that her lips—not her green eyes, contrary to what others might think—have a special something that constitutes her trademark. And the Chicago native, who says her lips *never* get chapped because she routinely nurtures them with petroleum jelly topped off with the prettiest glossy lip colors, finds that even when asked during photo sessions to communicate with her eyes, she can't help but do so through her lips, which she says "comes easily and naturally."

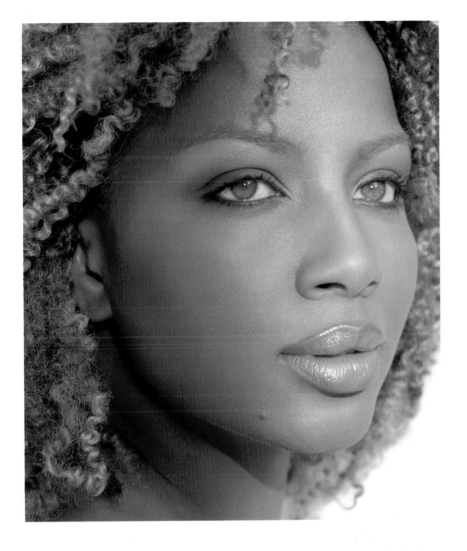

Model
Wyinnetka Aaron

To keep your lip appeal intact and serve great style, keep the following in mind:

- To protect and treat lips, always use a balm with SPF 15 or higher and such antioxidants as vitamins A, C, and E.

- If lips get flaky, heal them with a lip product that contains smoothing alpha-hydroxy or salicylic acid.

- Don't let a cold sore ruin a really important day. See a dermatologist to have it injected with a dose of cortisone to take down the swelling, and then conceal it with makeup, using a sterile cotton swab.

- Have fun with texture when experimenting with lipstick—from sheer stains to moist mattes and tones, from sensuous nudes to luscious color.

- Try mixing textures. For example, layer loose shimmer powder over lip balm and under a sheer gloss—so fab!

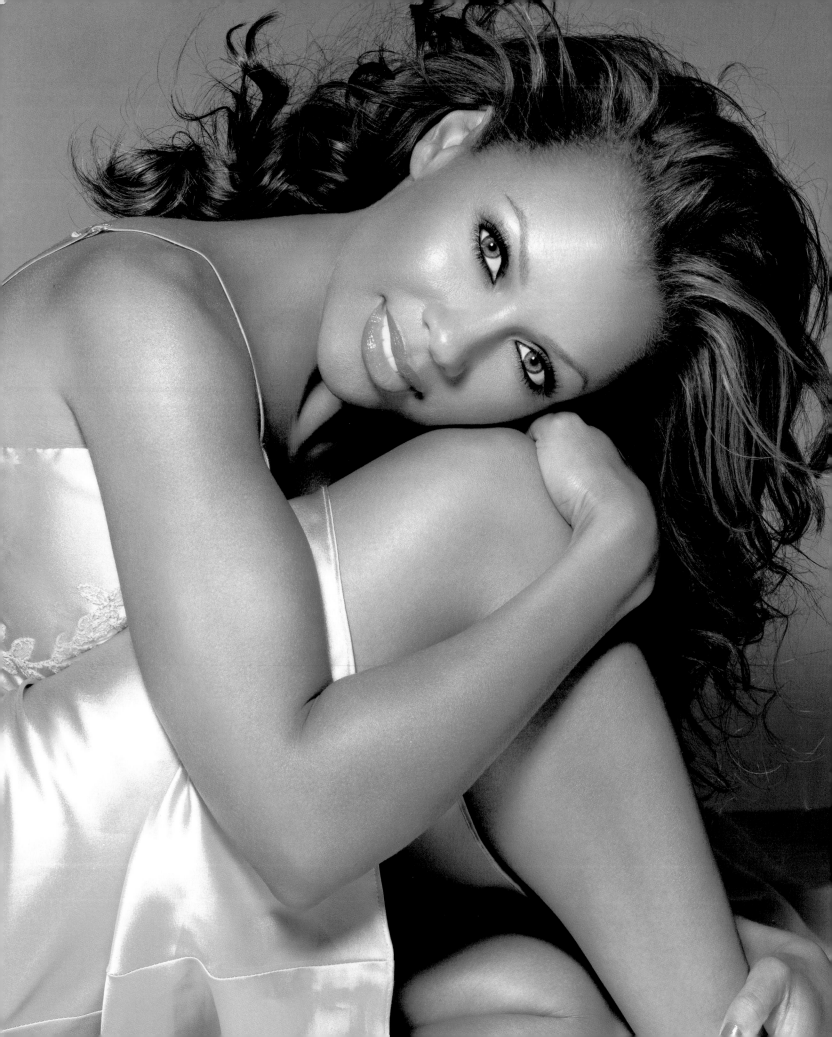

Work Iconic Legs

Grammy winner Patti LaBelle will tell you in a heartbeat that she derives the most fun expressing her beauty by "gleaming up my legs, wearing no stockings, and letting them talk for themselves!" Says the former track runner, "I always knew it was my legs. They were always strong, and running track—I was a really fast runner—helped to build them up and shape them." For LaBelle, who loves showing them off during her soul-stirring performances, high heels and a slit sure to please are musts!

To give yours a glam finish with superstar shape appeal, put the following into play:

- Exfoliate dead skin at least once a week with a hydrating body scrub. You can make your own with one cup of brown sugar and half a cup of baby oil, or mix brown sugar with an inexpensive body lotion to formulate a creamy paste. Massage in a circular motion, moving up the legs from feet to buttocks, and rinse.

- Get hair-free with a professional waxing or a depilatory aimed at coarse hair.

- Always moisturize legs while still damp, and try a bronze-tinted body lotion or cream for a lovely sheen.

- When baring legs after a long winter undercover, begin using a self-tanner for deep skin tones a few days beforehand to affect the look of legs on a summer vacation!

- To tone, take the stairs (two at a time) whenever possible instead of elevators or escalators.

- To sculpt, go for squats, lunges, and pliés.

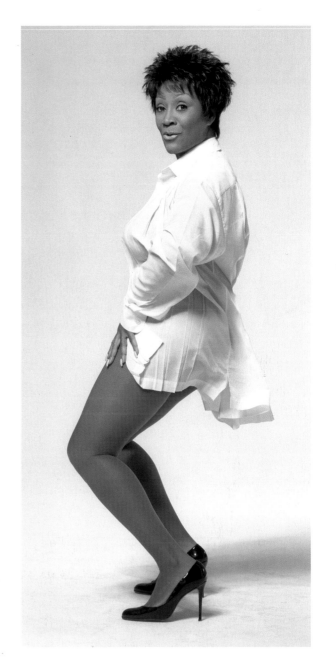

OPPOSITE:
*Singer and actress
Vanessa Williams*
ABOVE:
*Singer
Patti LaBelle*

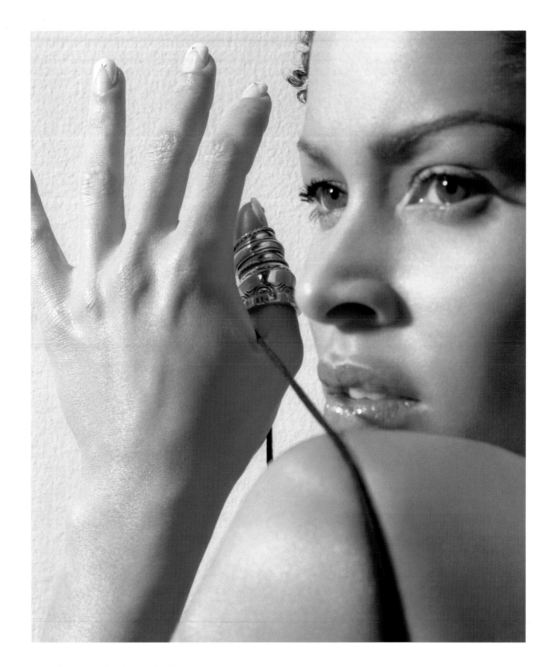

SELF-SEDUCTION

Nail a Look, Hands Down!

It goes without saying that a model's hands are always in the spotlight. Rochelle Hunt, who was discovered on the beach in Anguilla at age eighteen, has been a favorite hand model of mine for nearly ten years. Aside from her perfect nail beds and always smooth cuticles, I find her to be especially in touch with her hands in the way she uses them on camera—probably due to the fact that she's also a guitarist. Hunt, who works a signature look when she's out of the spotlight, credits her lovely hands to her parents, as well as to "keeping them manicured and not cutting my cuticles," which results in painful peeling.

Model
Rochelle Hunt

Give yourself a hand while nailing great style with the following maneuvers:

- Keep moisture in the flow and an even tone by using a hand cream with antioxidants, sunscreen, and one or more of the following: hydroquinone, kojic acid, or glycolic acid.

- Exfoliate hands weekly and have paraffin treatments whenever possible.

- Use cuticle oil routinely. For extra coddling, apply petroleum jelly and cover with white cotton gloves as a skin-softening overnight treat.

- Frequent hand washing can dry skin out, as can the use of quick-drying antibacterial agents designed to kill germs on the spot. To protect hands, use a water-resistant lotion with silicone and petrolatum, as they form a protective veil over skin.

- Help scars heal while they're fresh and lessen your chances for scarring with over-the-counter silicone sheeting bandages.

- Get rid of unsightly veins through sclerotherapy or treatment with the intense pulsed light (IPL) laser.

- Go for the unexpected on nails—switch up the classic French manicure with surprising shade mixes and textures, or add charm appeal with minute adornments that say you.

9

The Art of Picture-Perfect Beauty

"It is the decisive moment!"

Henri Cartier-Bresson, Photographer

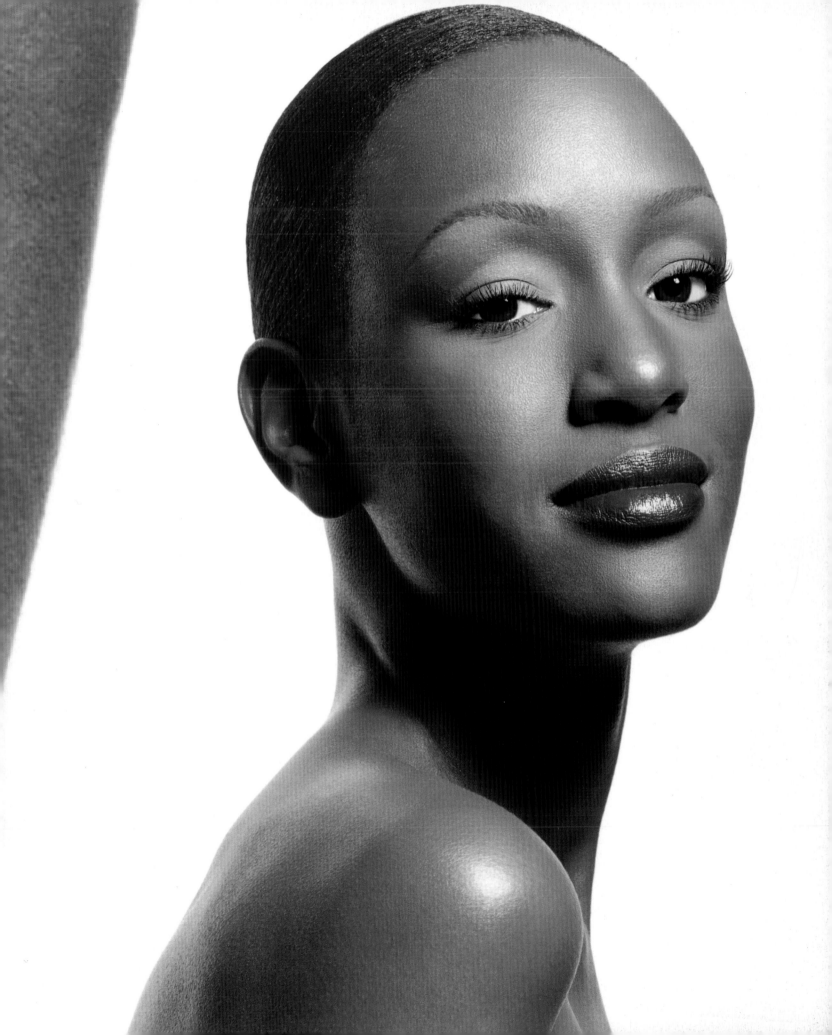

To me there's always been something quite magical about photography. Perhaps it's because my mother placed it on a higher level, both personally and professionally, that I came of age having such great respect for this most intriguing form of self-expression. Our house was filled with framed professional portraits, informal snapshots, glossy photo albums, and even a few newspaper clippings bearing paparazzi images of my mother and the beautiful people whose world she was a part of. On a professional level, there were backstage snapshots of beauty under way, fine composite shots, and album covers of the Divine One, singer Sarah Vaughan, whose look my mother played a key role in as hairdresser, makeup artist, and wardrobe stylist, ensuring an image that would befit one of the greatest jazz vocalists of all time. What I found fascinating about it all was how every picture spoke volumes about the person portrayed, almost allowing the viewer an intimate glimpse of their soul, or at the very least another facet of the person within. And yet inasmuch as the images gave the viewer this revelation, I later came to see that the very process of taking a photograph was often a major tool of self-discovery for the subject. Herein lay a world where you could evoke the personas of your desires and intensify the dream through hairstyling, makeup, fashion, even the setting. Why, in the hands of a good photographer you could be anyone you wanted to be!

By the time I entered my teens, I had become acutely aware of this through the many American as well as European fashion magazines my mother kept up with. What I noticed about them all, aside from the always confident gestures and incredible clothing the women wore, is that many of the same models were featured, and yet, depending on the publication, they took on a different aura from issue to issue—sometimes from page to page—within the same publication. And this is when I really learned to appreciate the art form of photography. One day while I was still in high school, my mother brought home a magazine that stood apart from all others. This one was especially for me. It was called *ESSENCE*, and it made its mark the moment I saw it, for it was full of the most striking Black women I had ever seen! Why, I was swept away, for it was like a dream you could touch. There were women of all shapes, flaunting their beauty through all types of hairstyles, makeup with no apologies, and bare brown skin that made you *so* love the idea that the Creator had given you some of this! Soon after, I made up my mind that I wanted to become a model, and through my mother's help I began learning the ropes of this highly competitive profession. One day I paid a visit to the magazine's headquarters on what's known in the industry as a "go-see." It was like walking into a *happening*. There in a little townhouse (the magazine's offices at the time) were visions of Black beauty, both adorning the walls and up and down the aisles typing the last word on style and substance! And then I met Susan L. Taylor, who at the time was fashion and beauty editor, and *nothing*, as they say, was the same. Thirty-two years later, I remember it as one of the most affirming experiences I've known. She was, to quote an old expression, "large and in charge," and I immediately loved her for it. Not only was she in command of her *space*, but she was in full possession of herself, confident, radiant, and with that same generous spirit she possesses to this day.

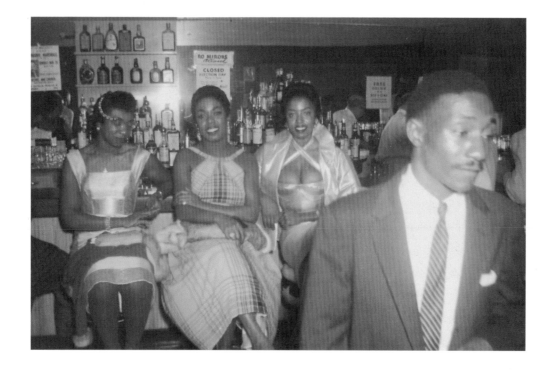

THE ART OF
PICTURE-PERFECT
BEAUTY

FAR LEFT:
*Modina Davis Watson
and* (MIDDLE)
*legendary vocalist
Sarah Vaughan*

Later my dream came true and I realized the honor of gracing the magazine's fashion and beauty pages. It was this experience on the other side of the camera that taught me the value of what goes into a good photograph. But it wasn't until I became an editor that I fully grasped what makes a *great* photograph, which without a doubt is one that captures a moment that you'll want to remember or indulge in forever.

Today, with twenty-three years as an editor and thousands of images behind me, I can tell you that whenever I step into the studio I'm on a journey to capture a *great* photograph. I've been taught by one of the greatest mentors a person in my position could have in this business: Susan L. Taylor, who encouraged me to dream and to dream big. Her goal was always to surprise, and with that came a constant push for the unexpected. With this being my daily bread, it wasn't long before I found the courage to go as far as my creativity could lead me, all the while working in tandem with the many talented sisters and brothers who've had their say in the look of the magazine's testimony known as *ESSENCE*. Now whenever I step into the studio, more often than not I've visualized the shot in my mind way before I arrive on the scene. By that point, the dream has come together simply by putting the right creative team in place to execute it. And since I'm clear that the camera captures more than what meets the naked eye, I'm prepared to spend a good deal of time fueling the mind of the subject being photographed so she can step confidently into the moment, because therein lies the wellspring! I've worked with many of the world's most iconic models, from Pat Cleveland, Beverly Johnson, and Iman to Naomi Campbell, Tyra Banks, Karen Alexander, Alek Wek, and a host of others so dreamworthy I could not even begin to have a say-so about them within the confines of this space. And yet to this day, my greatest delight of all continues to be found in working with celebrities or in doing beauty makeovers with real women. That's because I'm always looking to crystallize a side of the subject that the world—even they themselves at times—have yet to see. Quite honestly, I think of discovery, especially self-discovery, as one of the greatest joys there is. One of the best compliments I ever received about the work I'm involved in came indirectly from the queen of hip-hop soul, Mary J. Blige, who said during a radio interview shortly after her July '99 cover for *ESSENCE*, "I look like the woman I aspire to be."

What's really interesting is the fact that no matter who the subject is—whether it's Kimberly Elise, the young actress who first stole our hearts in *Beloved* and then again in *John Q* and who more than surrendered to the process of sun-kissed makeup, wispy eyelashes, and lots of gleaming to her beautiful brown skin for the January 2001 cover of *ESSENCE*, or Queen Latifah, who allowed us to express hand-combed hair, a naturally glamorous take on her makeup, and a rather playful side of her for the January '98 cover—the idea of discovering a look that's entirely different has always been a key element. The success came about from the subjects' confidence and their desire to push the envelope. Many times it was truly a case of acting, really sinking deep into a role and ultimately ending up with an image that stood out as *the* shot. On the other hand, there have been those times when a shoot was most difficult. Those were the times I deemed as "nobody home," meaning there was no one at home inside for us to work with and challenge! Those were the shoots that from the beginning were "a wrap," as we say in the industry, because they yielded nothing but the same buttoned-up images and plastic smiles that one can find in any camera shop. There were also times when I've stepped into the studio and the celebrity just wasn't comfortable having a picture taken at all. Those were the days when I wondered how someone could be so at ease making a movie or a video and yet not possess this same energy for a photograph. Since that time I've come to the conclusion that photography asks a lot more of its subjects. First of all, it asks them to *get still*, and that's something some of us just aren't comfortable with. We've become so accustomed to keeping busy or to knowing life on the move that getting still makes us irritable because we don't know what to do with ourselves. Sometimes, according to the experts, this can also come from what's known as "spiritual poverty." And the camera, or the idea of sitting for a photograph, makes us uncomfortable because it seemingly peers too closely. In the end, we become edgy or vulnerable because the process makes us feel exposed, as if the camera is able to reflect what lies within. But truth be told, we need to do the self-examination and then attend to what's lacking there—not for the sake of a photograph but in order to become all that we need to be.

As celebrity photographer Matthew Jordan Smith puts it, being comfortable with yourself is key to the process. "Getting to know yourself, love yourself, be yourself, allows you to relax and let down all the barriers," says Smith. A large part of that lies in doing the inner spiritual work that's critical to self-appreciation. We attend to our bodies every day, but often our spirits go lacking. That's unhealthy. So it's important to perform that "inner checkup" so you can get to that place where you're more than comfortable in your skin. Do so by acknowledging what's going on within and then make it a point to release whatever it is that doesn't edify you, because you can't use it! Remember, confidence is a virtue that you should be in full possession of, and it comes by way of knowing what you bring, loving it, and then continuing to affirm that knowledge daily, so that

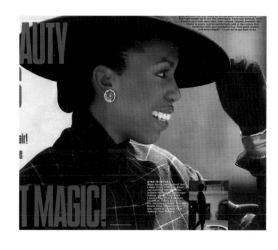

Mikki Taylor, 1978, as she appeared in ESSENCE *magazine*

THE ART OF
PICTURE-PERFECT
BEAUTY

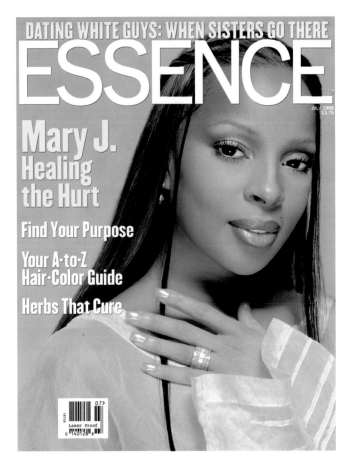

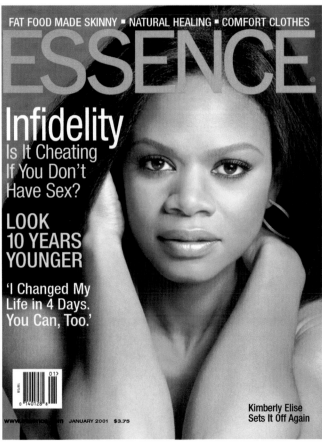

whether you're in front of the camera or just stepping out in the world in your day to day, you're clear about what you possess. I heard singer and poet Jill Scott tell a crowd one evening, "I know I'm fine—I was born fine! My grandmamma was fine, my mama is fine, and so I don't have any trouble believing it!" Now that's affirmation!

When you stand in front of a camera with that kind of confidence, you *want* to deliver. And you know what? The very idea of taking a picture becomes a fun, exploratory experience. When you think about it, there's so much more to all of us than meets the eye—in fact, I say there are many women inside each of us. So each time you take a photograph you should be ready to show your stuff.

Therein lies another reason why I really love celebrity shoots, particularly those where we've "got game," meaning the celeb comes in ready to travel and experience something greater than she may ever have imagined. For example, I've worked with Halle Berry on several *ESSENCE* covers, and to her credit, no two have been alike. Whether on location in the desert or in the close confines of a New York studio, she brings a refreshing, "why not?" energy to the set and steps into the zone instantly. And I really don't think it's because she's an actress as much as it is her confident approach to life and her clear sense of self. Ditto for

Tina Turner, who came to the studio for what was to be a two-hour shoot for the magazine and turned it into a six-hour marathon, dancing and having the time of her life throughout the session. And I don't think I'll ever forget that epic sitting where eight of Hollywood's top actresses came together for what was truly an extraordinary session filled with so much love and spirit that every shot was frameworthy. To this day, I marvel at that May 2000 cover, for it displays a group of sisters truly at home with self and more than ready to let the world know that this is what it looks like! Then there was that legendary cover of Oprah Winfrey back in June 1991. That too was a magical moment. I don't think anyone had ever seen Oprah barefoot before, let alone ever so sensuous—after all, we weren't used to seeing TV personalities that way, especially someone as prominent as Oprah! Nonetheless, I went in search of Oprah the woman, and I wanted to break some barriers—the way I saw it, we had already featured her as a talk-show host on a previous cover, so here was an opportunity to show another facet of her. I remember thinking how important it was to capture her relaxed, intimate, and in a way that said "I'm *so* comfortable with me." That's why in the end, shoes got in the way, lips had to be soft and dewy, and her hair had to be glamorous with a capital G! "*ESSENCE* was the first to say, 'You're beautiful, you're somebody special, you're worthy,' and to see myself as a big, full-bodied, full woman, fulfilled—that was an extraordinary moment for me!" says Oprah. The team and I were spellbound that day, because she went all the way from doing the proper breathing that generated the most serene face for the camera to relaxing into the position and serving great body language. Watching her was like witnessing a vision unfolding before your eyes. To this day, that cover remains one of my favorites, because not only did she step into the moment, she took it over the top, making it the frame of a lifetime!

For certain, a lot goes into a great photograph, but the essential ingredient is the subject and what she or he brings to the table. Just look at young

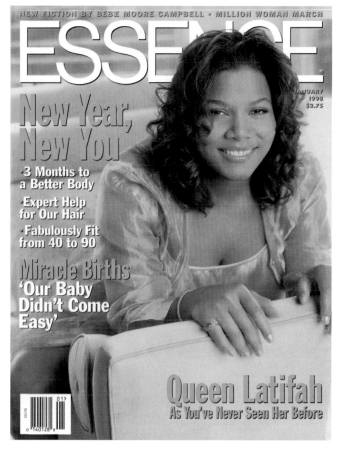

Rapper and actress Queen Latifah

THE ART OF
PICTURE-PERFECT
BEAUTY

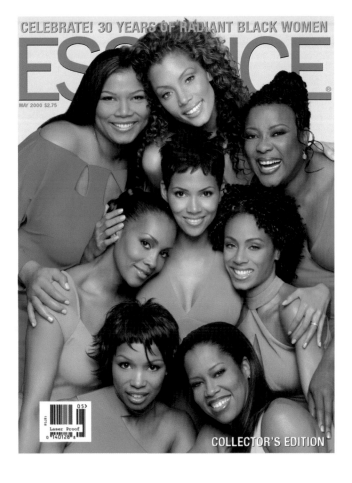

Aladrian Crowder, pictured on the opening spread to this chapter. Crowder was on her way to being a freshman in college when she sat for this image, which became *ESSENCE*'s August 2000 cover. She didn't bring hours of experience behind the camera into the studio that day. What she brought was her own refreshing confidence and an open mind! This was all we needed to capture a moment in her life where she was on the threshold of a new beginning. That is precisely why I think photography is one of our greatest mediums for recording all that's fabulous about us. It has been a form of documentation central to Black life in America since it began. Every time you attend your family reunion, you're able to sense what your elders and extended family were like, just from those framed images that were so lovingly preserved. When you look at your great-grandmother or aunt, you're able to glean their beauty, style, and personality traits. Without these precious images, many of us wouldn't know who we are and the legacy that we've been handed. Oh yes, the stories that our mothers and fathers are able to recount have their place, but believe me, it's the photographs that help to make them real! When I think about all the times my mother would go to have her portrait taken or have a photographer at the house to shoot us, I'm more than grateful. Ditto for those snapshots that someone took the time to capture. Today these images— although few in number due to a house fire that claimed most of our treasures— are a source of remembrance and fortitude for me. For though she as well as my grandmothers and others are no longer near, I have a few precious images of all that they were still with me and am able to share them with my children and the generations to come. Therein is another reason why we need to bring this significant practice back into our lives. I see this as part of our responsibility in the journey of life. It's not just about us as individuals, but how we motivate and inspire those we touch, who will continue to build upon the legacy we ourselves are a part of. And we have to count this simple practice important. More often

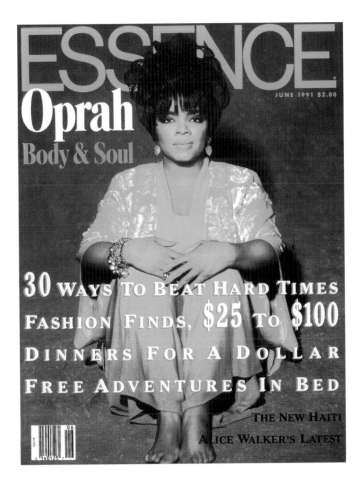

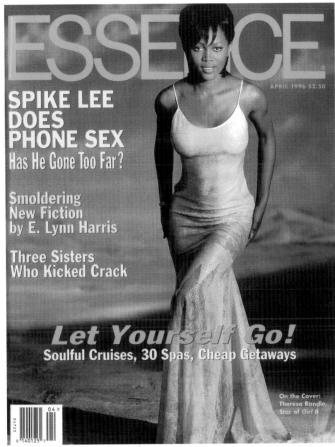

than not, many of us aren't in possession of a current photo of ourselves. And sadly enough, when a need arises for one, we're left trying to come up with something suitable. Moreover, unless we're part of an organization that routinely has its membership photographed professionally, the last portrait we have taken may be from our school days. I think we should take matters into our own hands and value ourselves and the joy of self-expression important enough to be captured in a professional photograph—more often than not. By this I mean that if you haven't sat for a portrait in more than five years, get it scheduled! Begin by making the necessary preparation to ensure that you end up with an image that begs to be framed. Rest assured, both you and your loved ones will be so glad you did.

OPPOSITE, CLOCKWISE
FROM TOP LEFT:
*Actresses
Queen Latifah,
Michael Michelle,
Loretta Divine,
Jada Pinkett Smith,
Regina King,
Elise Neal,
Vivica A. Fox,
and Halle Berry*
ABOVE LEFT:
*Talk-show host and
actress Oprah Winfrey*
ABOVE RIGHT:
Actress Theresa Randle

Your Best Shot!

Believe it or not, taking a great photograph lies more in your hands than it does in the person behind the camera. In fact, what I know to be true above all else is this: If you want to end up with an image that sweeps you off your feet, make it a practice to live your life in a way that affirms and honors you, both within and without, and you'll make it happen every time. Another essential primer that ensures great results is conceptualization. Simply taking the time to sit down and make those all-important notes about what you want is key. That alone will put the control in your hands where it belongs. Think about whom this image is for, where you'll place it in your home, and who else will receive this dynamic image of you as a gift they'll treasure. "If you're taking this portrait for your mate, that's a different aesthetic from one that you might take for your family," says New York–based fashion stylist Malissa Drayton Lisbon. A close-up for your significant other might have a more playful or romantic energy and capture you in a more intimate light and setting, whereas a portrait for the family will more than likely feature you in a more formal light and offer a completely different persona. What I've learned from communicating with photographers and creative teams over the years is that it helps to bring along materials that give evidence of what you're looking for. Whether you pull images from magazines or photos of those you love that bear the kind of feeling, lighting, or any other details that appeal to you, this is a very important step that will move you just that closer to getting what you want from the end results. "Ultimately," says Dawn Haynes, of the Dawn to Dusk Image Agency, an L.A. organization that sets up glam teams to make artists such as Halle Berry, Shemar Moore, and Nia Long feel and look their best, "it's important to be able to say, 'This is what *I* want out of the shoot.'"

Essential Elements for a Dynamic Session

Clearly preparation plays a great role in determining how fabulous your image will turn out. As an editor, I spend weeks discussing everything from concepts to just who will be a part of the creative team that will ensure the results we're after. This always looks at the subject being photographed and includes such details as what attitudinal qualities should be showcased, what's key about their beauty, and, at the end of the day, what the overall image should say. The first time we photographed model Naomi Campbell for an *ESSENCE* cover, it was all about capturing her voluptuous lips and her insouciant sass! To do so, I had the makeup artist capture the full-blown beauty of her lips in pure red. Without a doubt, she brought the attitude! For actress Theresa Randle, it was all about her striking confidence and toned, hourglass figure. She was photographed on a faux desert set, wearing a gorgeous body glove of a dress to showcase her whittled waistline and washboard abs.

Once a concept is determined and any feature points are highlighted, then it's time to select the photographer, makeup artist, hairstylist, and wardrobe stylist to execute the project. There are times when a prop stylist is also part of the team, whether to locate one special chair that will allow the subject to get cozy and really give up the energy desired or to find just the right fabrics to add a bit of color and texture to the overall look. To me, these are the essential elements for a dynamic photo session. For you that means giving careful thought to the look you want to communicate and then going about the business of just who should be a part of the team that's going to ensure that you shine. Maybe your session should take place in your home, where there is that special chaise or love seat. Perhaps your current hairstylist is just the one to deliver the look you want on camera; on the other hand, you might want something totally different for your shoot, and therefore it may mean challenging your stylist to offer you something other than what he or she is used to creating. Trust me on this—creativity is essential to the game and often plays a greater role than you think in delivering the fascinating as opposed to the mundane. In this case, you might also have to look beyond your regular stylist to achieve what you want. For example, if you desire to be photographed in the most intricately designed braids and your stylist isn't an expert braider, then that means you need to reach out to someone who is. It's worth doing the homework, however, as it will pay off by giving you the look you desired and a photograph that captures you in a way that expresses your spirit in this season of your life.

It's also important to secure a professional makeup artist who knows how to give good face on *us*. Many of you have checked in with me to secure some of the talent *ESSENCE* uses, and yes, they are available to you. However, if you find that their rates include travel and accommodations that compromise your budget, don't stop there—ask their bookers when or if they're headed your way and schedule the sitting accordingly. Or ask them for a recommendation, as they often have talent in other cities or colleagues who, though not well known, are quite skilled and available to you at a more affordable rate. Another alternative is to look to cosmetic lines based on the approach of professional makeup artists. More often than not, they feature special events at their department store counters, when they bring in professional artists to help savvy women like you learn new techniques and experiment with texture and color. This is your opportunity not only to increase the skill of your own hand but to discern what you like and what you don't as well as network and meet *the* makeup artist who can create the

EXPERT SHOPPERS

Tapping into a personal shopper can be easier than you think. While appointments are preferred, most are available to assist you with a minimum amount of notice. Just remember this complimentary service is meant to simplify your shopping experience and ensure that you're a completely satisfied customer. So if you're contemplating a photo session (or simply have an occasion where you need to look your ultimate best), check out the resources listed below for the ultimate style advice:

- **Nordstrom: Personal Touch. Call 800-695-8000 for your nearest location**

- **Macy's: Macy's By Appointment. Call 800-343-0121 to locate a store with an MBA program near you.**

- **Marshall Field's: Select personal shoppers program. Call 800-695-0275 to locate a shopper in your area, or log on to www.fields.com**

- **Henri Bendel, New York City. Call Michael Palladino at (212) 373-6353 or e-mail him at mpalladino@limited.com.**

look you want on camera. A word of caution, though—be careful when it comes to relying on a makeup artist who works with a portrait photographer, because they usually have a limited selection of shades that'll work for us. If you do find that this is your only option, then take such essentials as foundation, powder, lipstick, and lip liner along with you.

Finally, there's the subject of wardrobe direction. You don't need me to tell you how important this component is, but I will say this: Don't compromise! Make it a point to work with someone who not only understands fashion but, more importantly, gets your style and what you want to communicate so that when it's time to sit for your image you don't find yourself distracted by the clothing. For sure, this is an area that can make you feel totally fab or highly uncomfortable, so do the homework. Begin by looking to the personal shopper at your local department store as a great resource, as my friend Bonnie McDaniel did when she started having herself photographed. Bonnie, who today is in the public eye both as an author as well as an advice columnist on family relationships for Fox Television, continues to find this approach most successful, as it helps her to feel and be herself, as opposed to communicating a style at odds with who she is. What's key to being assured you've found the person who understands you best is the interview process. By all means come prepared with those details about your style that will be significant to the session as well as questions about the colors and silhouettes that will flatter you best. And here I say keep an open mind. Moreover, don't take a lot of folks along with you—confine it to that one person you trust, as too many opinions will ruin your decisions and turn a fun experience into a ball of confusion! In addition, know that the personal shopper should have questions for you that point out your likes, dislikes, and figure concerns as well as those that give him or her an idea of how you're going to be photographed—for example, whether you'll be sitting or standing, and other such pertinent elements as the lighting and the environment or background.

If you find that all a particular personal shopper really is about is pushing the clothing, just thank him or her for spending the time with you and move on quickly! However, once you're convinced that you've found your expert, follow his or her advice and make the investment on pieces that will make you feel good not just for the photo session but for any special occasion, and extend your wardrobe to boot.

Finding Your Best Angle

When we were growing up, there were times when our friends would accuse us of being a "show-off." Other times they'd say, "She thinks she's so cute!" Truth be told, they were right! If you think about it, at those particular times in your life you had a fierce sense of self and were about the business of expressing it to the hilt. You knew what worked and how to pull it off, and you delighted in flaunting it. Today it's simply called "self-awareness," and you know what? Everyone wants it! But all kidding aside, self-awareness is one of the key elements needed to capture your personal flair on film. And while we've examined this a lot through the previous chapters, unless you're used to being in front of a photographer on a regular basis, it's fair to recognize that there's an added dimension to translating it for the camera, particularly from a physical perspective.

Matthew Jordan Smith, photographer and author of *Sepia Dreams*, a celebration of Black achievement, reminds us that "being aware doesn't mean being tense. In this case it really means being conscious of your body language." One way to get to know yourself is to have a practice session in front of a mirror. Call on those familiar gestures that you love (you might even discover some new ones), but just really relax and get into it. Make it a point to discover the difference between what you like and what you *love* when it comes to your posture, how you're positioned, and how you come across overall, all the while keeping in mind how *you* want to be captured in this portrait. Practice sitting, standing, maybe even lying on the floor, so you'll know just where you feel—and, equally important, come across—most comfortable. It has been said that in our mind's eye we all have a stronger side; when you're practicing, see if you find this theory to be true. Perhaps you'll discover different characteristics about both sides that you want captured during your photo session. Either way, becoming aware of yourself in the mirror will give you a clear picture of what you want to express, and it will up your confidence as well. From there, keep an open mind and trust the photographer you've chosen to lead you into new territory. You'll both know what works and what doesn't. What I've learned over the years is that no gesture is too small when it comes to a photograph. Sometimes a subtle message is sent by the way the head is lifted, or the slight tilt of a shoulder serves to turn an okay image into one that's quite wonderful. When you're in the flow, one great expression or gesture leads to another. Many of the images of this book came from a series of expressions. Notice I didn't say *poses*, which I believe is the most unnatural thing on earth! In fact, over the years I've gone on record as telling women not to model or pose in front of the camera. If it isn't a real gesture or expression of the moment that conveys a certain truth and is therefore ever so compelling, skip it! And I encourage you to do the same, because at the end of the day that's not the reality of who you are, and it's not how you should want to be remembered. Enough said!

Relaxation Techniques

Finding a comfort zone in front of the camera is different for everyone, but I can tell you that the kind of preparation mentioned previously will go a long way toward putting you at ease. What also helps is coming in with a mind-set that's completely ready and intent upon enjoying the process, something I really can't put enough emphasis on. Veteran portrait photographer Dwight Carter, who has captured some of the most riveting images of famous African-Americans in the last twenty years, sees this as key and takes it a step further by encouraging his subjects not to be too serious and to look upon having a photograph taken as an experience. According to Carter—who, by the way, feels it is his job to help subjects relax before the camera—another key is *not* to concentrate on taking the photograph. "Everyone's so concerned about what they're going to look like in the camera, when the real focus should be on emoting something wonderful," he adds. To me, therein lies one of the greatest relaxation techniques of all time. Often when I'm in the studio and a subject is having a little difficulty taking her mind off the camera, I'll step in and paint a scenario that really transports his or her mind to another place and allows them to work the feelings associated with the vision. I call this "visionary daydreaming" and find it so powerful that I used it as a tool for my daughter while she was giving birth. During the labor phase I took her to an imaginary beach and helped her to view the birthing pains as waves that would come and go. Since she was hooked up to a monitor, I could tell her when the contractions—the waves, so to speak—were coming in, when they were at their height, and when they were moving out. Her role was to breathe during the process and focus on the waves, not the pain or how long before the baby would arrive. In the end, this proved to be a far more pleasant experience for her because of where she placed her focus, and thus she welcomed her baby daughter in a calm and relaxed frame of mind.

Fashion stylist Malissa Drayton Lisbon also cites the importance of taking an imaginary journey as a relaxation tool during a photo session. Says Lisbon, who's worked on many magazine and publicity shoots, "The process of letting your mind take you somewhere dreamworthy during the sitting can really take away the edge of putting yourself on display."

What also helps you to relax is encouraging feedback. During the many shoots for this book, I watched the subjects unfold as photographer Paul Lange fed their spirits with the most empowering responses to what they were serving before him. I believe that in the end it made them want to go on to higher heights in every instance. To say they enjoyed the process is an understatement. One look at Patti LaBelle's image and you know she's gone beyond merely having a picture taken and is completely in a zone—feeling good and freely singing and dancing from the heart. To look at Oprah is to know that she is totally at ease and loving every nuance of that sunny, breezy moment! Looking at these images, I can still hear Paul's enthusiasm as he's moving in and out, clicking away: "Yes, Oprah, that's it, you're all the way there, don't move, I love it when you lift your eyes there," or "Come on, Patti, go for it, you're wonderful, absolutely right on!" I can't imagine that anyone would find it hard to relax and feel good with such moving encouragement. So be sure to talk with your photographer beforehand about this essential communication, which will help you to relax and achieve the image of your desires.

Most importantly, free yourself up about the entire process. When I'm in the studio working on a cover, I often remind myself and the team that all we need is *one* great shot! So be at ease—you have everything you need to come away with that and more. From there, follow these proven tips to help you relax during your photo session:

- Routinely take deep breaths in through your nose and out through your mouth during those periods when the photographer is reloading the camera.

- Periodically roll your head from shoulder to shoulder. Shrug your shoulders up and let them go to release tension and relax your upper body.

- Get up and walk around every now and again so that you can return to the set calm and refreshed.

- Stay in the zone. Forget the cares and responsibilities of the day and really allow yourself to be completely absorbed in the experience at hand.

- Keep a positive frame of mind. Don't allow yourself to dwell on any perceived limitations—there are none!

- Make sure you have music on hand that both lifts and relaxes your spirit.

Communicating with the Camera

Watching a photographer and subject at work is not unlike observing two people engaged in a dance. There's movement, spontaneity, and (for sure) an electrifying chemistry! And what I've found to be true more often than not on the best photo sessions is that the subject is in the lead! No mystery there—as I said previously, when you know yourself, you're clear about what you bring. Nevertheless, I will admit that translating this before a total stranger can be a bit daunting at first. But rest assured that if you approach it with the right mind-set, you'll move beyond your fears and find yourself wanting to give more than you ever imagined.

Begin by keeping your perspective. Remember, this is *your* story that's being told before the camera, so don't try to be or play anyone else but yourself. This is your time to shine and express that special truth about you. Again, one of the easiest ways to sum it up for the camera is to simply look in the mirror, emote, and identify how you want to communicate. And while you're at it, really play it out, from a confident smile to a good laugh. Find your romantic side, get a bit playful, try for your more daring characteristics, or get as serious as you want to be taken. Then decide just what aspect you want to reveal in your photograph.

Once you're comfortable there, trust it. Most all of the experts agree that it's an honest emotion that makes for a memorable image you'll want to treasure. "It's not about a photographer forcing something onto you; this is your photograph, and you want to be remembered as you really are," says photographer Paul Lange. So go the distance by sharing what you want to communicate with your photographer, and let it be his or her challenge to help you reveal these aspects naturally.

On the other hand, though, there is something to be said for alternative ways to get at the image of your dreams and still keep it real. For example, if you find that you just can't connect with the photographer, you might try substituting someone you love for the photographer in your mind's eye and imagine communicating with that person instead. Of course, thinking about whom the image is for will help shape what you communicate as well. What won't work is having them present at the shoot! Believe me on this—the smaller the number of people present at a photo session, the more you'll be able to focus and really achieve your goals. In fact, many photographers not only discourage having other people there but will go as far as to block off the set so that they can maintain your full attention, thus preventing any distractions that could turn the photo session into a miss. Recognize that this is in your best interest, and wait until you have the film in hand to invite family and friends to have their say!

Finally, know that one of your best gauges on communication is to ask to see a shot periodically during the session, so you can see how you're coming across. From there, feel free to talk candidly with your photographer about those aspects that you especially like as well as any that may concern you.

This Is How We Do It!

There's no mistaking a great image—you know it when you see it. For models, photographers, and celebrities alike, achieving one comes by way of clear direction, by not being afraid to have a bit of fun, and through trust. What you want to keep in mind is this: Always be true to yourself and what you want to express. Here, then, is the last word on what's essential to communicating in front of the camera and getting the shot of your desires

> "Loud, funky, hip-hop music and a great photographer
> who really knows when he or she has gotten the shot!"
> **PATTI LABELLE, SINGER EXTRAORDINAIRE**

> "Take a deep breath and look like you're comfortable
> with yourself and the world."
> **IMAN, COSMETICS ENTREPENEUR**

> "Trusting the photographer and making sure they treat you like a lady!"
> **VANESSA WILLIAMS, SINGER, ACTRESS**

> "Let go of inhibitions and let yourself shine!"
> **SHAKARA LEDARD, MODEL AND ACTRESS**

> "Be yourself, like you're ten years old again
> and have faith in the people around you!"
> **KWAKU ALSTON, CELEBRITY PHOTOGRAPHER**

> "Relax. Don't force a smile. Don't put on too much makeup!"
> **VERONICA WEBB, MODEL, ACTRESS,**
> **AUTHOR OF *VERONICA WEBB SIGHT:***
> ***ADVENTURES IN THE BIG CITY***

> "Don't put on a front. What you hide is the most is obvious,
> so don't try to be something that you're not—it never works that way.
> Even if people don't get who you are at first, pretty soon they'll get you,
> because if they feel like it's coming from a truthful place, they'll feel
> connected to that truth, because the essence of who we are is truth
> and they'll get the connection sooner or later."
> **BRANDY, SINGER AND ACTRESS**

Believe it or not, I'm more than finicky about having my picture taken! Every detail, from just whom I'll trust behind the camera to who will do my makeup, is of major production status to me. That's probably because I'm so close to it all. On the other hand, it really has a lot do with the fact that images are about defining a moment and capturing someone's innermost expressions, so it's essential that the experience of it be one that sweeps me away! After all, if I'm going to deliver, then ultimately there must be something in it that makes me want to go the distance! This is something that I try to ensure for everyone that I've ever worked with. Feeling as passionate about the experience as I do moved me to come up with a few checkpoints (see below) for communicating on camera in the form of quips that I share with subjects when I'm in the studio. I have found they make subjects appear not only as though they have mastered the art of being photographed but also as though they are completely enthralled by the experience. Trust me—once you put them into play, your images will have everyone asking, "Is that you?"

Smile, You're On!

Bust to the sky! Nothing kills a great photograph quicker than poor posture! If you're sitting, be sure to sit up tall, press your shoulders down, and yes, lift your bust proudly to the sky.

Part your lips ever so slightly and breathe in and out through your mouth. No question, this one takes practice, but it releases the tension in your face and allows you to divert some of your focus away from the intensity of the photographer and the camera. When combined with pleasant thoughts, you won't fail to look absolutely amazing!

Keep that bright look of expectancy! If you really want to take a memorable photograph, this is it. To do so, simply fix your eyes on the camera and think of it as a door through which someone that you're dying to see is going enter at any moment. The key here is keeping the excitement both in your eyes and on your lips. And don't let the feeling get stale—turn away from the camera as often as you need to so you can find the freshness of this expression again and again.

Think! Oftentimes I'll tell the subject, "I need to know what you're thinking," because they've gone blank and aren't emoting anything worth capturing. Don't let this be true of you—it's important to translate a range of emotions for the camera, as this both keeps the photo session exciting and in the end makes for far more interesting choices in the film. So whether it's a degree of flirtation or simply a knowing look that says total confidence, make sure you keep your thoughts engaged and focused.

The Art of Taking a Fine Portrait

There was a time when the concept of a personal portrait was a very set thing, unless of course you were involved in the arts. With few exceptions, the subject was posed and always formal in demeanor. But times are changing, and more and more you're apt to see women captured in a way that's reality-checked and approachable. To me this is a direct reflection of the times we live in, the influence of the media, and the overall casualization of America, whereas everything is a lot less structured than it used to be—from when and where we eat to how we dress in the workplace. It's also reflective of how we feel about ourselves. Take, for example, the portraits in this book. They all testify to the wonder of our truths: owning our lives, confident about our beauty, challenged but nevertheless triumphant, and on purpose. Why, even the rituals shown or alluded to make up the reality of our lives. This is the new page in our history, and to me it is not a question of whether it should show up in a photograph, but how!

Finding a photographer who gets this and can translate it into a great image is paramount. Word of mouth followed by a careful examination of the photographer's work is a good place to start, unless of course you desire to take the route of magazines and ad agencies and engage a commercial portrait photographer. Either way, what's critical to getting the shot of your desires is setting up an appointment to talk with the person who may end up capturing *your* image. Make sure you come away feeling confident that he or she is the one. According to Matthew Jordan Smith, "a good photographer is one who can bring out the best in you." In order to do so, he believes, the photographer should get to know as much about *you* as possible. Smith, who admits that taking a photograph is a very personal experience, makes it a point to find out such details as the kind of music his subjects like, their food preferences, and what kind of environment makes them comfortable, so that by the time they're in front of his camera, they're ready to open up and trust him for a great image.

Keep in mind too that this is a commitment that you've made, and only aim for the best. And remember, you get what you pay for, so be sure to educate yourself about the qualities of a good photograph. "While a lot of what you're seeing in a photograph can be considered subjective," says Lange, there are some aspects that aren't. So when you examine a portfolio, Lange advises critiquing it against the following basics:

- Are the images sharp?

- Are they lit well? Or do they appear dark or overexposed?

- Is the light flattering? Or does the subject's skin tone appear gray or ashy?

- Does the subject look comfortable?

- Is the composition of each photograph flattering to the person pictured?

- Does the background complement the subject? Or is it harsh, unflattering, overpowering?

Says photographer Dwight Carter, who recently photographed author and poet Maya Angelou, "If you don't like the way other subjects appear in their book, there's a chance you won't like the way you look either!" So it's important to examine the work closely so you won't end up being unhappy with your image. And I urge you to really pay close attention to the lighting. Nothing compromises an image like poor lighting. I can tell you from years of observation that lighting our brown skin is no small feat for even the most expert photographers—I've see some of the best have to work it out and even rethink some of the things they were sure of! To ensure that you're truly satisfied, take the advice of those in the know and request a warm light, as opposed to a cool one. Lange himself is a strong believer in the use of gold reflectors—large metallic boards used to reflect light onto the skin—for us instead of silver or white because the last two cast an ashy hue. "Even the light source should bear a degree of warmth and sparkle," he adds, and therefore he never uses a dull white umbrella to light us sisters (at least not without a gold reflector), preferring those that are metallic-lined to give our skin a sensuous glow. On the other hand, you might decide to have your image captured outdoors; if so, know that the best time to do so is when the light is beautiful and golden, which Smith says is at sunrise or sunset.

Backdrops or backgrounds also play a key role to the overall image. If you look at most magazine covers or image-driven profiles of celebrities, you'll notice that the backdrops are simple and clean, unless of course the subject is photographed in an environment such as their home. This really allows the subject to shine. It also helps the magazine to share more cover lines or attention-getting copy—critical features in the publishing war going on at the newsstands today! The lesson to be derived here is this: Don't go for anything gimmicky. Avoid at all costs computerized backgrounds and anything that appears the least bit overpowering. Keep to what is fresh and simple and, most of all, complementary to your skin tone. Look to shades of gray, soft white, or warm neutrals. And be sure to have yourself photographed with black-and-white film as well—you'll be surprised at how it equalizes everything and really puts *you* in the spotlight.

Finally, remember that everything you and the photographer have given thought to—because this is a collaborative effort—should show up in your image.

For certain, those things that you've missed will too. So make it a point to be involved in every facet, including the technical, and by all means don't be afraid to ask questions about anything and everything you want to know.

Ready for Your Close-up?

No matter what you want your image to convey, taking the right approach to makeup, hairstyling, and wardrobe is essential to getting there. Here you want to think like the pros and have it all mapped out in advance. That means having an informative dialogue with everyone involved as well as scheduling important grooming appointments central to a polished image. Fashion stylist Dawn Hayes makes sure her clients have a facial, manicure, pedicure, and any facial waxing done ahead of time, so that the temporary redness that accompanies these processes can subside. Says Hayes, "We also have them get a colonic to make their eyes white, and above all else, get a good night's sleep so they show up on set vibrant and glowing!" Most importantly, do whatever you need to do to put yourself totally at ease, from arriving early to bringing your personal grooming essentials and any foundation garments that are going to give the clothing the fit you desire. Now you're ready for your close-up!

Makeup 101

For sure, makeup is an individual form of expression, but here too there are some guidelines to follow that will ensure yours is picture-perfect. Makeup artist Jay Manuel, who routinely steps into the studio to turn out Tyra Banks, singer Mya, and Iman, believes that what makes a great portrait is "clean beauty"—in other words, simple makeup with a particular focus on the finer details. "Curl the lashes and go for more mascara, groomed brows and a seemingly clean face—that way you stand out more," he urges. Makeup artist Sam Fine not only concurs but encourages us to get to know ourselves and what works and what doesn't on a very personal level. Says Fine, who works the look of singers Mary J. Blige and Brandy, "Makeup enhances the beauty that you already are, and the success of it begins by loving yourself and then choosing the right things to express it, carefully." All in all, it's best to not overdo, for in the end, this misstep will read loud and clear on film.

What's important to the process is allowing the proper amount of time so neither you nor the makeup looks rushed! So you should figure on an hour for expert makeup. I've noticed that a lot of that time is spent enhancing the model's skin with foundation, powder, and perhaps bronzing powder to add warmth and dimension, since everything tends to lighten up or wash out in photography. As women of color, our faces are not monochromatic. More often than not, that's why many of us don't care for foundation, because it makes our skin look flat and unnatural. When prepping one of us for a professional photograph, a skilled makeup artist will make sure not to lose the subtle nuances of our skin tone so that we don't end up looking masklike or overly made up. For Fine, this means shading the forehead or framing the face with bronzer. It also involves perfecting our canvas as a primer for this stage by using concealer a couple of shades lighter under the eyes and to cover blemishes and minor scars before foundation so that the overall look is free of any unwanted shadows or dark spots.

In addition to this basic priming, makeup artists also spend time on the little details that really distinguish a look, such as bleaching and/or filling in the brows and perfectly lining the lip so there's depth but no telltale dark liner. Perhaps capturing your style for the camera will involve blending one or more lip colors or textures to achieve it precisely. Or maybe your emphasis will be on the eyes, and that might entail some subtle sculpting using neutral browns to accentuate their shape without adding color. Experts tell us that for most great portraits, the eyes really command one's attention, which is why, when it comes to makeup, less can be so much more. Take my advice and avoid heavy shimmers, which have a tendency to blast their presence on film due to the lighting. Ditto for dramatic color—don't do that to yourself—you'll be over it before you view the film! According to Manuel, the use of top liner is another don't, because it creates an abrupt line that diminishes the eye. "It's better to curl the lashes and use lots of mascara, which will make the eyes appear more open, cleaner, and younger," he adds. However, if you find that liner is a personal beauty staple, try rimming the eyes with a warm brown shadow to cleverly create depth without a hard edge. This is why I encourage you to engage a professional makeup artist, because technique really can make or break your shot. So go for it and prepare for the process by knowing that you're more than worth it. "Think of this time as a ritual that will help you rest and relax and come out looking fabulous," says Fine. Finally, keep this advice in mind from Darryl Johnson, L.A. fashion stylist and costumer for such powerful films as *Boyz 'N the Hood* and *Scary Movie:* "The soul of a moment is always in the face, so make sure that it's as beautiful as you want it to be!"

Here are some dos and don'ts that'll make sure you're in the know and camera-ready:

DO

- Correct any discoloration with a concealer

- Aim for a second-skin finish by choosing the proper foundation shade and formula

- Look to a soft cream or powder blush or a bronzing powder to subtly warm the cheeks

- Apply loose powder with a large brush to set makeup, pressed powder (with a large powder puff) sparingly for touch-ups

- Aim for a natural brow that's well groomed; use a brow pencil or powder to fill in any sparse areas and subtly enhance shape

- Curl your lashes for lift and separation

- Use two coats of mascara and comb through lashes after applying to remove any clumps

- Blend a bit of foundation onto your lips to cancel out discoloration before applying lipstick

- Line lips for definition, using shades that are browned; pay close attention to the outer corners—top and bottom—and blend, blend, blend

DON'T

- Apply makeup without first using a moisturizer

- Use fingers to apply base; always use a makeup sponge

- Forget to blend foundation onto your neck and chest when wearing an open neckline, so everything matches both in tone and in coverage

- Use concealer without foundation

- Overpowder—it'll build up and appear unnatural

- Try bright blush tones—they're as far from natural as it gets!

- Utilize products sold as "contour," as they tend to be ashy and unnatural-looking

- Fail to touch up often, particularly to cancel out shine in the T-zone, to remedy creasing underneath and above the eyelids, and to refresh lip color

- Exaggerate or overextend the shape of your brows

- Attempt to use black to line your lips

Hair Dos and Don'ts . . .

Think beautiful, simple, and timeless as your guideline to a great look on camera. Here the experts really caution you to stay away from trendy dos that will date your image. Follow this advice even if you're trying a styling technique that's separate and apart from the look you normally wear. From there, put the emphasis where the pros do and concentrate on those details that will ensure a polished finish on film. If your hair is relaxed, that means paying special attention to the edges, ensuring that they're smooth and that the ends are trimmed and appear nice and shiny. For natural hair you should keep a close watch on any errant locks and frizzing. Master stylist Derrick Scurry, whose natural dos rock the runways in Milan and Paris, often wraps the ends of the hair around a small curling iron to produce a smooth, frizz-free finish that'll last. Using an anti-frizz agent from root to ends is also helpful. To Annu Prestonia, stylist and owner of New York City's Khamit Kinks, a natural hair salon, another caveat is to have any specialized styles—such as braids, twists, or knots—executed so they are technically correct from the roots to the ends and that any partings are absolutely precise. She adds, "Any style that's not stationary is going to move, especially if it touches the shoulders, so working with a professional stylist on set to make sure your hair looks perfect from roll to roll is a must."

Hairstylist Oscar James, who clips and styles actresses Halle Berry and Vanessa Williams, believes proper prepping is foremost to a great portrait. He cites such steps as a great cut, roller-setting for fullness, and the use of styling aids that add body as important measures for relaxed tresses. Like many stylists in the know, he'll also go the distance to give fine hair additional support by working in some pieces. There are also times when he'll work in added hair for highlights, depending on the photographer's lighting, especially if the subject's hair is very dark. I've found this to be a great technique, particularly because our hair, in its deeper hues, tends to absorb light, which is why the use of shine products is really important on set. I've seen photographers struggle to light our hair to keep from losing the styling details as well as our unique textures on film. So check the image before the photographer goes into film, and if you're not able to ascertain those characteristics, ask for an adjustment to the lighting so you can.

Once you've made your decision concerning the look that's right for your image, aim to keep it soft and touchable, unless it's a stationary style such as cornrows—and even then try to keep to the same principle, which may be as simple as choosing human hair over synthetic for your extensions and leaving the ends free to curl. If you're the kind of sister who wears a signature style where every hair is in place, have your stylist try a hand-combed finish for certain areas or go for less curl on camera so that the hair doesn't look too done. If you wear bangs, maybe go for a look that's more fringe than blunt and doll-like. For natural hair, make sure your stylist goes easy on the use of any styling aids with a wet finish, such as a thick holding gel—it'll show up on film, and it won't be cute! And keep in mind that shape and texture are everything, so don't be afraid to finger-comb or rod-set your hair in its natural state, especially if you wear twists or locks.

Ultimately, the last word on the perfect do centers on the proper tools and styling aids for final touch-ups at the studio. Here is a prep list from the pros:

- Conditioning mousse (without alcohol)—to create fullness, give hold (relaxed hair)

- Light styling gel—for smoothing, soft hold

- Pomade—to smooth stray edges, control ends

- Light holding spray

- Sheen spray

- Scissors—to clip strays

- Blow dryer—to release tight curls (if necessary)

- Flat iron—to smooth or shape (as needed)

- Curling iron to bump ends

- Velcro rollers—for a quick set if hair is too flat or lacks body

Style Basics

If I could tell you only one thing about your on-camera look, it would be this: Make sure that whatever you choose to wear not only looks good but (equally important) *feels* good! If you look at most of the clothing selected for *Self-Seduction*, you'll notice that we worked with a great deal of knitwear, from cashmere to cotton. This was not only due to the wonderful clean lines that are always the basis for a great portrait, but also because fabrications such as this offer up what I call a "feel-good factor" that I think should be essential in anything that touches a woman's body! When I sat down with Pamela Macklin, who served as our style director, and our core team for this project, we made it our goal to showcase the sisters being photographed and to not have the clothes become so important that they would be a distraction, both to the subject and to the end results. To her credit, the term *timeless* became the direction we would all cling to when it came to the selection of clothing for these images. Ditto for the use of solid tones, which yielded a fresh palette of neutrals—from white to black that would work well against our skin tones. Thus the real focus centered on what we were trying to communicate in each of the images, as well as determining the unique assets of the women being pictured. All of this was meshed together in concert with the backdrop and lighting so that everything would be in complete harmony. This is the kind of hands-on approach you want to take when it comes to your portrait.

To make sure your wardrobe selection is on point and camera-ready, photographers and stylists alike recommend the following:

- Keep your clothing selections simple, timeless, and monochromatic.

- Avoid anything trendy, patterned, or ornate, as it will immediately claim *your* spotlight!

- Put your emphasis on a great neckline, such as a V-neck, a scoop neck, or an off-the-shoulder or face-framing line, and on good fabrics that retain their shape and finish.

- Make sure your garments fit properly and are steamed to perfection

- Be sure to keep jewelry to a minimum, as too much jewelry or pieces that are too important can overpower as well as date your image.

Finally, unless yours is a formal corporate portrait, I say *please* defy all notions of getting dressed up! Make looking great on camera effortless by giving thought to what you want your image to convey and then approaching it with what I call a "casual-luxe" feeling in terms of the clothing you select. By this I mean easy pieces, in the most luxurious fabrics, that communicate your style to the letter. Again, by working with a pro you'll remove the guesswork from the selection process and easily achieve your goal. For Macklin, who knows fashion both from a retail perspective as a manager and from her work behind the camera for print and TV media, the trade secret to a great photograph comes down to this: knowing yourself, expressing your assets, and finding your comfort level within the clothing. When these checkpoints are satisfied, she adds, "you can stand in front of a camera and deliver the beautiful—yourself!"

How to Capture a Winning Snapshot

Wedding photographer and model Regina Fleming captures the most awe-inspiring images of brides and grooms on their special day that I've yet to see. What I love about them most is that they're like stills from a movie—frozen in time, yet with all the exhilaration and joie de vivre of the moment! This is exactly why I caught up with her to learn what makes a great snapshot, because I believe the elements that make any one of her photographs are the same for yours. Here's what you need to know:

"The perfect photograph is one that captures your spirit. It shows your personality, and people know who you are when they see it. It offers some type of emotion from you, whether happiness or laughter, but it should pull something from you. So the answer to getting a great snapshot is being ready! And be sure to breathe, because if you don't you get that deer-in-the-headlights syndrome. Think of the camera as a long-lost friend you're happy to see. And remember that your eyes are the most important part of a photograph—they show your soul—so think great thoughts!"

One could say there's a real art to taking a photograph; however, I'm convinced, as are the people who stand in front of or behind the camera every day, that the greatest key to all of it lies within. I asked West Coast photographer Steve Williams, who captures celebs on the red carpet at every turn, to tell us just what he thought was the most essential thing to remember to for a winning photograph, and this is what he had to say: "You want to come off calm and cool and collected and let the spirit of God in all of us just demonstrate who you are!" Enough said.

Works Cited

Bailey, Diane Carol. *Natural Hair Care and Braiding* (Albany, N.Y.: Milady Publishing, 1997).

Copage, Eric V. *Black Pearls: Daily Meditations, Affirmations, and Inspirations for African-Americans* (New York: Quill, 1993). Quote from Kwame Nkrumah.

Fletcher, Barry. *Why Are Black Women Losing Their Hair?* (Seat Pleasant, Md.: Unity Publishing, 2000).

Heart and Soul Magazine, *Healthy Living Journal.* Quotes from Ntozake Shange, Marian Wright Edelman, and Jewel Diamond Taylor.

Newman, Richard. *African American Quotations* (Phoenix, Az.: Onyx Press, 1998). Quotes from Mae Jemison, Nikki Giovanni.

Photo Index

All photography by Paul Lange unless otherwise indicated; style direction, Pamela Macklin; photo session coordinator, Sandra Martin

Cover Subject: Karen Alexander; Agency: IMG, New York City; Makeup artist: Roxanna Floyd, Illusions, New York City; Hairstylist: Keith Campbell, C.O.I. Studios, Brooklyn, New York; Manicurist: LuLu; Stylist: Elaine Wallace; Slip: Cristina Perrin

Page iii Subject: Randy Graves; Agency: Willhemina, New York City; Hairstylist: Derrick Scurry, www.derrickscurry.com; Makeup artist: Roxanna Floyd, Illusions, New York City

Page xiv Subject: Oprah Winfrey; photo by Paul Lange "© Harpo, Inc., 2002. All Rights Reserved"; Hairstylist: André Walker; Makeup artist: Reggie Wells; Sweater: ELM Designs

Page 8 Subject: Susan L. Taylor; Hairstylist: Ellin LaVar, LaVar Hair Designs, New York City; Makeup artist: Nzingha Isis Gumbs, The Z-face; Sweater: ELM Designs

Page 15 Subject: Jennifer Thread McHenry; Hair: Derrick Scurry, www.derrickscurry.com; Makeup artist: Lanier Long

Page 16 Subject: Jacqueline Peters Canon; Hairstylist: Diane Bailey, Tendrils Wellness Salon for Natural Hair, Brooklyn, New York; Makeup artist: Lanier Long; Sweater: ELM Designs

Page 23 Subject: Oprah Winfrey; photo by Paul Lange "© Harpo, Inc., 2002. All Rights Reserved."; Hairstylist: André Walker; Makeup artist: Reggie Wells; Sweater: ELM Designs

Page 25 Subject: Randy Graves; Agency: Wilhemina, New York City; Hairstylist: Derrick Scurry, www.derrickscurry.com; Makeup artist: Roxanna Floyd, Illusions, New York City

Page 39 Subject: Star Jones; Hairstylist: Oscar James, Ken Barboza Associates, New York City; Makeup artist: Jay Manuel, Ken Barboza Associates, New York City; Manicurist: S. Michele Echols; Prop stylist: Malissa Drayton Lisbon

Page 47 Subject: Sadie Delany; Photo courtesy of Daily News Pix

Page 51 Subject: Lisa Butler; Agency: Paulines, New York City; Hairstylist: Derrick Scurry, www.derrickscurry.com; Makeup artist: Christopher Michael, Ken Barboza Associates, New York City; Manicurist: LuLu

Page 63 Subject: Cynthia Bailey; Agency: Wilhemina, New York City; Makeup artist: Roxanna Floyd, Illusions, New York City; Manicurist: Rachel Garielov, Mark Joseph Salon, New York City

Page 67 Subject: LaTanya Richardson Jackson; Hairstylist: Oscar James, Ken Barboza Associates, New York City; Makeup artist: Roxanna Floyd, Illusions, New York City; Manicurist: Tamika Hardy, www.@cty-nyc.com; Sweater: ELM Designs

Acknowledgments

All good and perfect gifts come from above. I give thanks and praise to Almighty God who enabled me to author this message of love supreme. I give honor to my ancestors whose strengths laid the foundation I now build upon, especially my maternal grandmother, the late Bessie Boyd, who was my leaning post, and to my paternal grandmother, the late Maggie Graves, who gave me an appreciation for the simple things in life that money cannot buy. Thanks to "Grandma" Clara Watson, for the courage to be herself and live by her own code of ethics; I am empowered to this day by her example. Thanks to my sister Candace, for being there every day in every way with love, prayers, and the encouragement I needed in both high and low times! Thanks to my sister Deborah for setting such a rich example of what it means to be a good mother and a woman who remains steady in the journey. Also, thanks to all those who have touched my life in countless ways and helped me to grow. My deepest thanks go out to: Anita Diggs; Maureen O'Neal, Allison Dickens, Barbara Greenberg, and the team at Ballantine for their belief and support of this project; my legal team headed by Allen Arrow, and the diligent help of Ivan Saperstein and Jonas Herbsman, for their wisdom, guidance and care; the researchers, whose conscientious help and attention to detail, has meant so much: Delora E. Jones, Pamela Edwards, Stephanie Scott, Barbara Brandon-Croft; special thanks to Paulette Brown for her tenacity and excellent assistance with photo research and permissions; Julia Chance; Victoria Benning, Nancy U. Hite, Gayle Williams; Ashley Taylor; Sharon Elcock, for your encouragement, and assistance with agency credits; Michelle Webb of The Ideas Co., for strong support and belief in this project and for encouraging yours truly in the good and adverse seasons of the journey; Jennifer Lange, Nancy Trefny, and the team of photo assistants: Christopher Mello, Julian Bernstein, Eric Vogel, and Matt Coch of 1313 Photo Arts Ltd.; the superb managers who made the improbable happen: Vince Cirrincione (Halle Berry)—you went the extra mile and I am deeply grateful; Stephen Jensen (Patti LaBelle), Ward White (Erykah Badu); Lisa Shannon (Tyra Banks) and the publicists who played such a vital role, Patti Webster (Patti LaBelle), Gina Avery (Vanessa Williams), Marvet Britto (Vivica A. Fox), Serena Gallagher (Erykah Badu); special thanks to Libby Moore, Amanda Casgar, Lisa Halliday and Deb Olson of Harpo Productions for their excellent and diligent help; and personal assistants and those who helped secure time to share: Ayeola Johnson (LaTanya Richardson Jackson), Amanda Wessels (Star Jones), Lorraine Krich (Iman); the many empowering women and men who strengthened us from the start and/or through the journey, many just by their presence and gifts of the spirit: Dr. Eugene Lawton, Sister Diane Lawton, Author Terry McMillan, Johnny Gary, Malissa Drayton Lisbon, Jenyne Raines, Ms. Debra Parker, Gayle King—three cheers for your beautiful spirit! Roxanna Floyd, Angela Burt-Murray, Sam Fine, Oscar James, Keith Campbell, Derrick Scurry, Christopher Michael, Brother Clifton Thomas, Jackie Putman, Sandra A. Martin, Avis Yates, Diane Weathers, Barbara Britton, Enedina Vega, Elayne Fluker, Jennelle Mahone-Sy, Elaine Wallace, Claire McIntosh, Bridgette Barlett, Vanessa Bush; Tony Moschini, formerly of Sun Studio for your special belief in this project and the enormous time you gave of yourself to see that we had everything we needed—you're the best, let the record show! Special thanks to the Dakota Studio for making us feel at home. My deepest gratitude to the many experts who gave of themselves in support of women the world over—whose knowledge shall move us and the generations that follow fast-forward. Finally, to those whom I can't recall, God knows who you are and I ask that He shower you with His richest blessings for your goodness!

A One World Book
Published by The Ballantine Publishing Group

Copyright ©2003 by Mikki Taylor

All rights reserved under International and Pan-American Copyright Conventions.
Published in the United States by The Ballantine Publishing Group, a division of
Random House, Inc., New York, and simultaneously in Canada by Random House
of Canada Limited, Toronto.

One World and Ballantine are registered trademarks and the One World colophon
is a trademark of Random House, Inc.

www.ballantinebooks.com/one/

Book design by Joel Avirom and Jason Snyder
Design assistant: Meghan Day Healey

The Cataloging-in-Publication Data for this title
is available from the Library of Congress.

ISBN 0-345-44745-X

Manufactured in Italy

First Edition: April 2003

10 9 8 7 6 5 4 3 2 1